One Welfare

A Framework to Improve Animal Welfare and Human Wellbeing

One Welfare

A Framework to Improve Animal Welfare and Human Wellbeing

Rebeca García Pinillos
BVetMed, PhD, Dip (AWSEL) ECAWBM, MRCVS

With guest contributions

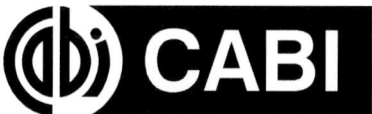

CABI

CABI is a trading name of CAB International

CABI	CABI
Nosworthy Way	745 Atlantic Avenue
Wallingford	8th Floor
Oxfordshire OX10 8DE	Boston, MA 02111
UK	USA

Tel: +44 (0)1491 832111
Fax: +44 (0)1491 833508
E-mail: info@cabi.org
Website: www.cabi.org

Tel: +1 (617)682-9015
E-mail: cabi-nao@cabi.org

A catalogue record for this book is available from the British Library, London, UK.

Library of Congress Cataloging-in-Publication Data

Names: Pinillos, Rebeca García, author. | C.A.B. International, issuing body.
Title: One Welfare : a framework to improve animal welfare and human wellbeing / Rebeca García Pinillos.
Description: Wallingford, Oxfordshire, UK ; Boston, MA, USA : CABI, [2018] | Includes bibliographical references and index.
Identifiers: LCCN 2017060812 (print) | LCCN 2017061261 (ebook) | ISBN 9781786393869 (pdf) | ISBN 9781786393876 (ePub) | ISBN 9781786393845 (hbk : alk. paper) | ISBN 9781786393852 (pbk. : alk. paper)
Subjects: | MESH: Animal Welfare--organization & administration | Intersectoral Collaboration | Global Health | Environment
Classification: LCC SF604.5 (ebook) | LCC SF604.5 (print) | NLM HV 4708 | DDC 636.08/32--dc23
LC record available at https: //lccn.loc.gov/2017060812

ISBN-13: 9781786393845 (hbk)
      9781786393852 (pbk)
      9781786393869 (PDF)
      9781786393876 (ePub)

Commissioning editor: Caroline Makepeace
Editorial assistant: Alexandra Lainsbury
Production editor: Marta Patiño

Typeset by SPi, Pondicherry, India
Printed and bound in the UK by Antony Rowe, CPI Group (UK) Ltd

Contents

Tables

Case studies and contributors

Reviewers

Section 1: Freda Scott-Park; Phil Arkow, Nuria Querol Viñas
Section 2: Gary J. Patronek; Frech Ochieng
Section 3: Charles Smith, anonymous Animal Welfare professor, Stella
          Huertas
Section 4: Sarah Heath, Anne Fawcett, Henrik Lerner
Section 5: Mike Appleby, Antonio Velarde, Peter Stevenson

Acknowledgements

Special thanks to all One Welfare 'team' contributors: Michael Appleby, Freda Scott-Park, Charles Smith, Antonio Velarde, Xavier Manteca and the One Welfare artwork designer, René Held, who have provided me with a combination of moral, technical and practical support since the beginning of this venture. Without you the concept of One Welfare would not have reached this stage and I am very grateful for your advice and ongoing support.

Thank you also to all of the case study contributors and peer reviewers who have really made a difference with their inputs, examples and very helpful suggestions and comments.

Many thanks also to those who have assisted selflessly with their advice and support through the past years, including David Grant, Mohan Raj, Elizabeth Kelly, Kate Sharpe, Derek Belton, Anne Fawcett, Don Broom, Lotta Berg, Sarah Heath, Jane Gibbens, David Montgomery, Zeev Noga, Nigel Gibbens and Tomás Fisac.

To those who attended the very first discussions and One Welfare stakeholder meeting that took place during 2015: your input, constructive challenge and comments at the preliminary discussion helped me mature and develop the concept into a full framework. Among others, my thanks to Javier Dominguez and John Lawrence, FSA; David Harris, APHA; Robert Huey, NI CVO; Sheila Voas, Scotland CVO; Simon Waterfield and Sue Ellis, Defra; Catherine O'Connor, Public Health England; Andrew Voas, Scottish Government; Irene Allen, Welsh Government; Sandra Dunbar, N. Ireland Government; Michael Seals, Animal Health and Welfare Board for England; Jessica Stark, World Horse Welfare; David Bowles, RSPCA; Michelle Beer, National Animal Health and Welfare Panel; Sean Wensley, British Veterinary Association; John Blackwell, BVA; Peter Stevenson, Compassion in World Farming; Clare Kivlehan, Dog's Trust; and Mike Appleby, World Animal Protection.

Thanks also to those who have shared their examples and comments at the different talks and poster sessions or through engagement on social media.

    Thanks to everyone who took part in the One Welfare framework consultation for the time invested in helping shape up the framework, your valuable examples, comments, suggestions and references; all of your responses have helped to build and shape this book. Many thanks to everyone who participated, including: Heather Bacon, Jeanne Marchig International Centre for Animal Welfare Education; Dritan Laci, Agricultural University of Tirana, Faculty of Veterinary Medicine in Albania; Crispin Caws; Roberto Becerra, Asociación Chilena de Bienestar Animal; Suzanne Rogers, Human Behaviour Change for Animal Welfare; David Mongomery; Dale Douma, Manitoba Agriculture; Anne Fawcett, University of Sydney; David Bowles, RSPCA; Miiamaaria Kujala, University of Helsinki; Lotta Berg, Swedish University of Agricultural Sciences; Satu Raussi, Finnish Centre for Animal Welfare; Laura Hänninen, Research Centre for Animal Welfare, Helsinki University; Franck Peron; Urs Lurcher; Elena Nalon; Paul Roger, Veterinary Consultancy Services Ltd; Emma Fàbregas, IRTA; Eleonora Nannoni, DIMEVET, University of Bologna; Eric Carrasco; Jenny Stavisky, Vets in the Community; Rahul Singh; Jorge Palacio, Universidad de Zaragoza; Nienke Endenburg, Faculty of Veterinary Sciences, Utrecht University; Raphael Guatteo; William Barker, Castle Vets; Amelia Garcia Ara; Laura-Jane Sheridan; Siobhan Mullan; Gareth Pearce; Barbara Schoening; Cristina Sobral, APMVEAC; Katia Di Nicolo; Christine Halsberghe; Good Dog Ownership School; Sylvia Masson; Amy Brown; Stephanie Presdee; Tanya Stephens; Marta Vieira; Wendela Wapenaar, University of Nottingham; David Oduori; Dorothee Krastel; Hen Honig; Donald Broom, University of Cambridge; David Morton; Harry Blockhuis; Michael Appleby; Daniel Mills; Pantaleo Gemma; Dovč, University of Ljubljana, Veterinary Faculty; Xavier Teles Canavilhas; Sira Abdul Rahman, Commonwealth Veterinary Association; Raquel Matos; Nick Saint-Erne; Sandra Carbonell; Morris Villaroel; Margarita Martin, Junta de Castilla y León; Shakira Free Miles, The SaveABulls; Paola van Dijk, van Dijk Veterinary Services Ltd; Sarah Cochrane; Gabor Bognar; Richard Rusk; Paul McGreevy, University of Sydney; Gustavo María, Universidad de Zaragoza; Ana Lucia Camphora; Beatriz Zapata, Universidad Mayor; Alma Vasquez; Ana Martos; Huw Golledge, UFAW/HAS; Jessica Stokes, Soil Association; Croatian Small Animal Veterinary Section; Gonçalo Da Graça Pereira; Carol Gray; Lewis Grant, VPHA; Karen Von Holleben, bsi Schwarzenbek, Germany; Jerry Aylmer; Zoe Belshaw; Martha Smith-Blackmore, Forensic Veterinary Investigations, LLC; Vivien Dillon; Warren Hidalgo Jara; Julia Clark; Yvonne Mackender, CAPB; Maria Reyero; Charlotte Burn, Royal Veterinary College; Claire Wade, APHA; Carolina Rosa; Rogerio Romeu; Camila Prado; Thais Santana; Helen Lemos; Gustavo Rezende; Ceres Faraco, Centro Universitário Ritter dos Reis – UniRitter; Osvaldo Silva, Pamela Andreia Chaviel da Rosa; Gabriela Freitas; Carlos Ellwanger; Carina Hullen; Aline Rossi; Ana Claudia Figueira; Les Eckford; Aida Garcia Pinillos; David Williams, University of Cambridge Veterinary School; Stella Maria Huertas,

Facultad de Veterinaria – Universidad de la República; Nat Waran; Neil Wedlake; Shane Ryan; Peter Wedderbun; Moritz van Vuuren, South African Veterinary Council; Belinda Johnston, Our Special Friends; Gary Jordan; Peter Watson; The Brooke; Ayssa Rahman; Rasto Koles; Charles Smith, The Farming Community Network; Sarah Heath, Claude Beata; Mohan Raj; Sandra Nicholson, University College Dublin; Hannah Buchanan-Smith; Branka Bukovic Sosic; Henrik Lerner; Macarena Vidal; David Grant; Belinda Nunes; Stephanie Torrey; Animals' Angels; Carla Molento, Federal Council of Veterinary Medicine, Brazil; SRUC; Gertie O'Rourke; Alison Hanlon, University College Dublin; Antonio Valcarce; Laura McAnea; Tasmin; Julia Havenstein Humphrey; Vicki Betton, PDSA; Marijana Vucinic; Al McLeod, The Brooke; Joan Lindenmayer, One Health Commission; Sophie Muset; Giuliana Miguel.

I have to also thank everyone who participated in the One Welfare framework webinar and the follow-up workshop meetings held in Defra and OIE as these final discussion sessions were crucial to refine the final framework and condense results that have now become a reality within this book.

Last but not least I would like to thank my family and friends who have been there when I needed to discuss the exciting, the good and the difficult times while developing the One Welfare framework and drafting this book.

Preface: A Note by the Author

The first time I mentioned the words 'One Welfare' was on 5 May 2015. I was participating in a meeting in Foss House, York, UK, on animal welfare at the time of slaughter, and trying to explain the relevance of multidisciplinary work to colleagues present. What appeared to be yet another intervention at a work meeting haunted me for days, as if by vocalizing these two words I unleashed a magical spell on me, which completely changed the way in which I would see things around my daily animal welfare role. Multiple interconnections flashed in my brain when discussing animal welfare topics and it then became clear to me that, while I and many other experts have worked on animal welfare for a number of years, we have yet failed to tackle many ongoing issues. My current thinking is that this is very likely to be happening because we have mainly dealt with animal welfare as an isolated issue, rather than as an integrated, multidisciplinary topic.

For some time I could not stop thinking about these two words and this led to discussions with some of my office colleagues, where I explained that I had a thought that could help us in our role to help improve not just animal welfare but also human wellbeing. My colleagues thought the idea sounded interesting and asked me to put my ideas down on a paper for discussion with the team. Shortly after this I circulated the first draft paper setting down the outline for 'One Welfare – a platform to improve animal welfare and human wellbeing'. The paper was very well received by colleagues and I was then asked to present this to the four UK Chief Veterinary Officers on 9 September 2015. At the meeting I presented my initial thoughts around One Welfare and the different suite of outcomes that derived from them. I was probed and challenged, with a very successful outcome. All four thought the idea was worth taking further, and shortly after I was asked to arrange a stakeholder meeting and present a proposal for the development of a One Welfare platform.

I organized the list of attendees, venue and date with the support of the Animal Welfare team in Defra. Attendees included a range of selected government departments, non-governmental organizations (NGOs) and veterinary organizations. The meeting took place on 26 October 2015. During the discussion some mentioned that the concept of One Welfare had in fact been mentioned by others in the past, although not in such a comprehensive way, with most focusing on particular aspects of the multiple ones described previously. All agreed that while it had been named, no follow-up work had really been done to develop it, and as a result it had not been widely adopted or taken forward. There was wide discussion around the concept and its possible outputs, as well as the overlap with the One Health concept. Some thought it would be best to focus on One Health, for simplicity; however, after the full discussion the majority agreed that having a welfare-focused platform could be a very useful tool to help improve animal welfare, human wellbeing and environmental goals. This would avoid the risk of notifiable disease and other health aspects taking over the welfare part of a single One Health concept.

It was not a government priority at the time to pursue this novel initiative but, as the stakeholder meeting raised very positive momentum, we agreed that I would continue exploring this concept privately on a voluntary basis. I then set up a private research initiative in collaboration with non-governmental colleagues, creating a new One Welfare 'team'.

I approached a number of stakeholders whom I knew had been undertaking One Welfare work through their careers. They included Mike Appleby, who through his role as a welfare scientist has produced and delivered many educational publications and talks related to One Welfare; and Freda Scott-Park and Charles Smith, who both successfully lead One Welfare NGOs: the Links Group and the Farming Community Network, respectively, within the domestic and farming environments.

We agreed to publish a letter to discuss the concept of One Welfare and invite others who had an interest and who had spoken or published material related to One Welfare in the past to join our team and take part in the full article we were preparing. This letter was published in the December 2015 issue of the *Veterinary Record* (García Pinillos *et al.*, 2015). A number of replies arrived, expressing an interest in participating and flagging up papers that had previously referred to the concept of One Welfare. It was in this way that we confirmed the absence of a cohesive approach and a fully comprehensive paper to cover this concept. After this I invited two further colleagues, Xavier Manteca and Antonio Velarde, who undertake key research and educational roles in animal welfare and One Welfare topics at international level, to strengthen the global focus of the project.

Following this I worked further on the draft paper I circulated in 2015, and circulated an expanded version to One Welfare team colleagues for comments and further input. The paper 'One Welfare – a framework for improving animal welfare and human wellbeing' was finally completed and submitted for publication. Given the unusual format and topic of the paper it was challenging to fit this into a scientific publication, and it was finally agreed that the paper would be published as a viewpoint within the *Veterinary Record*. The section stimulated much discussion and helped to further strengthen the topic.

In parallel to the above I worked with a volunteer professional designer, René Held, who helped in creating a logo and identity for One Welfare. This helped to build up a website, social media and almost a One Welfare brand that could be easily identified and recognized by anyone in the world.

After this, One Welfare took on a life of its own, with its own website, social media and international appearances. Support for the concept has not stopped growing ever since, and I am very grateful to everyone who has provided assistance and support along the way, towards the publication of this book.

The journey towards publication has helped me to explore further many domestic and global issues around the concept of One Welfare, and by doing this I have realized that One Welfare is already very much present in our lives and work. It is just that no one has named many of those activities, projects, publications, etc., in such a way before. One Welfare is already a reality and I am really hoping that this book will help to enable further development of existing and new initiatives to help achieve a better world for all.

Reference

García Pinillos, R., Appleby, M.C., Scott-Park, F., Smith, C. and Velarde, A. (2015) One Welfare – a platform for improving human and animal welfare. *Veterinary Record* 177(24), 629–630.

Foreword – Monique Eloit, OIE

The understanding and perception of animal welfare differs for each and every individual, region and culture. Animal welfare is a complex and multi-faceted issue, involving scientific, ethical, economic, cultural, social, religious and political dimensions. It is intrinsically linked with the environment and to human health as a whole. Increasingly we understand the connection and relationship between animal health, wellbeing and productivity to human health and wellbeing.

One Health is now well accepted as an approach to understanding the connections between human health, animal health and ecosystem health through interdisciplinary cooperation. In the same way, if we embrace the interdisciplinary approach in seeking to understand the contribution that animals make to well-functioning societies in different settings in the world, our understanding of the importance of animal welfare will deepen, as will our understanding of how it can be fully integrated into our animal owner-ship, husbandry and care practices.

Since 2002, when the World Organisation for Animal Health (OIE) spe-cifically brought animal welfare into its mandate, significant advances have been made in the development of science-based animal welfare standards, agreed by our 181 Member Countries following an inclusive engagement and adoption process. Science-based animal welfare recommendations have been codified in international standards for: transport of animals by land, sea and air; slaughter of animals and killing for disease control; produc-tion systems in various species; stray dog population control; use of animals in research and education; and working equids. All these are now part of the *Terrestrial Animal Health Code* and the *Aquatic Animal Health Code*. These provide essential guidance to OIE Member Countries to improve animal welfare and the wellbeing of their owners globally.

The OIE's role and processes for setting science-based international standards for animal welfare are now well established within the strategy and structure of the organization. But the OIE must continue to identify new thinking from scientific research, including research in social sciences, that can improve our standards development. During the 4th OIE Global

Conference on Animal Welfare in Guadalajara, Mexico, in 2016, and with the adoption the OIE Global Animal Welfare Strategy during the 85th OIE General Session in May 2017, the OIE has specifically acknowledged the importance of multi-stakeholder and interdisciplinary approaches to animal welfare, and integrated this into our work. We understand that we must continue to monitor and review our processes and standards, to seek new perspectives and new ways of viewing challenges, to ensure we are meeting the evolving demands of our members and the societies they and we serve.

In this regard, the OIE recognizes the importance of the new concept of One Welfare developed in this book, and welcomes its contribution to framing the many connections between humans, animals and the environment, and how harnessing this thinking will improve animal welfare. Our understanding of the concept will surely continue to evolve, incorporating a broad international view so that it becomes relevant to all OIE Member Countries.

Monique Eloit
Director General

The Path to Developing a One Welfare Framework

Introduction

The content of this book combines the result of personal ideas from the author and collaborating experts, stakeholder discussion outputs, published literature, participants to an electronic global consultation on a One Welfare framework and definition proposal, a global webinar and workshop-type meetings held at Defra and OIE, as well as a number of personal discussions and electronic exchanges with experts in related areas across the world.

Overall, the majority of discussions and exchanges have been extremely positive and supportive of the development of a One Welfare framework. Many identify this concept as a tool that would encourage and support collaborative efforts into work on the environment and on the health and welfare of humans and animals, while increasing public awareness of the connections that exist between these fields.

Many agreed that One Welfare is a concept that encompasses, in a multidimensional way, a number of areas, including:

- the problems of animal production, workers and the impact on the environment of livestock farms;
- the reduction of violence across the world;
- the connection between poor animal and human welfare states and how improved animal welfare can help improve human welfare.

Improvements in animal welfare do not always progress as expected and most of the time it is humans who cause the majority of animal welfare issues. It is therefore necessary to ensure that human welfare aspects are considered if we are to achieve effective animal welfare improvements.

Through the replies received during the electronic consultation it was clear that there are already a number of projects taking place across the world on the One Welfare orbit. There was also a strong desire for the concept of One Welfare to develop further, encouraging others to adopt similar ways of working and to create a platform enabling the provision of exposure and increased recognition of this work. A single concept connecting animal, humans, nature and their welfare appeals to many, and it is seen as something that will help expand many welfare projects and programmes – and launch new ones – for better animal, human and planetary welfare.

The One Welfare concept can help those working in veterinary practice and animal welfare organizations to understand and recognize the interconnections between their work, focused on animals, and wider society. It can highlight that the impact of their role goes beyond helping animals, and helps to stop suffering more widely, reaching humans and society. Many, in fact, might already have been working in this way during their careers, without naming the approach as One Welfare. In a similar way, this concept helps professionals working with humans – such as medics, nurses and social services professionals – to better understand the interconnections of their work with nature, including animals and the environment, and how working jointly with professionals in those fields can assist human wellbeing aspects in different ways.

One Welfare can assist individuals or societies, without a broad perception of the meaning of animal welfare, to fully understand the impact improvements in animal care can have and the different societal areas that relate to this. Some might say that this concept helps to take animal welfare to a new level of understanding, integrated within other disciplines within the One Welfare framework.

Respondents to the electronic survey included a number of professionals, such as:

- Those working in animal shelters, who understand clearly how their work relates to animal welfare, human wellbeing and environmental aspects.
- Officials undertaking farm inspections, trying to improve welfare standards in small production units. Some noted that they have used approaches akin to 'One Welfare' and found this to be an effective way of applying interventions. Officials also felt that One Welfare captures the spirit of their duty to society and future generations.
- Officials at slaughterhouses, who noted that improving animal welfare at slaughter would also help to increase respect for the staff, as in many places this is not a very valued job, despite being very challenging and difficult.
- Vets in practice, who acknowledged that they may come across human frailty in their clients, but are not often equipped to assist at this level, although efforts to build up support frameworks for domestic abuse, for example, are being set up.
- Animal welfare scientists, who were very supportive of the concept of One Welfare and see their role as key to increasing the evidence base on existing gaps.

There were, however, a number of relevant professionals in the framework who were less well represented and overall more difficult to engage with. These included medical practitioners, environmental and conservation experts; international development experts; criminal and legal professionals; and economists or social researchers. It is, however, hoped that with wider dissemination of the concept and increased efforts to establish collaborative work frameworks, the relationships between different professions will improve with time.

Fostering institutional interaction and empowerment is key to develop a One Welfare approach leading to more efficient outputs for all. Some countries lack this collaborative approach and the One Welfare framework can help identify relevant areas to their societies and provide some existing examples and references which can serve as a starting point on which to build.

Many see the connections made by One Welfare as a more efficient way to help tackle global problems, and have identified the value in developing further the evidence base in these areas. Embedding this concept within existing undergraduate, post-graduate and professional development in curricula has also been discussed, and some experts and institutions across different countries have already made a start.

One Welfare relates to sustainable and progressive coexistence of the planet's life forms. Dialogue and mutual respect are seen as essential to improve both the human and animal situation across the world, particularly in a context where humankind is the only species capable of consciously altering outcome paths.

Social responsibility and animal welfare improvements were key themes in several responses, where many wanted to be part of making our society and the lives of animals and our planet better.

Just as the physical conditions of humans, animals and the environment are interdependent, so is their welfare. The topic of animal welfare is still novel in many societies and sectors, particularly when compared with health, and has not been adequately explored in connection to human and environmental wellbeing. This book aims to assist readers in identifying these connections and to inspire them to continue building up the evidence base in this area by putting One Welfare into practice and documenting further examples of these connections.

Why Do We Need One Welfare?

The World Bank defines One Health as:

> A collaborative approach for strengthening systems to prevent, prepare, detect, respond to and recover from primarily infectious diseases and related issues such as antimicrobial resistance that threaten human health, animal health,

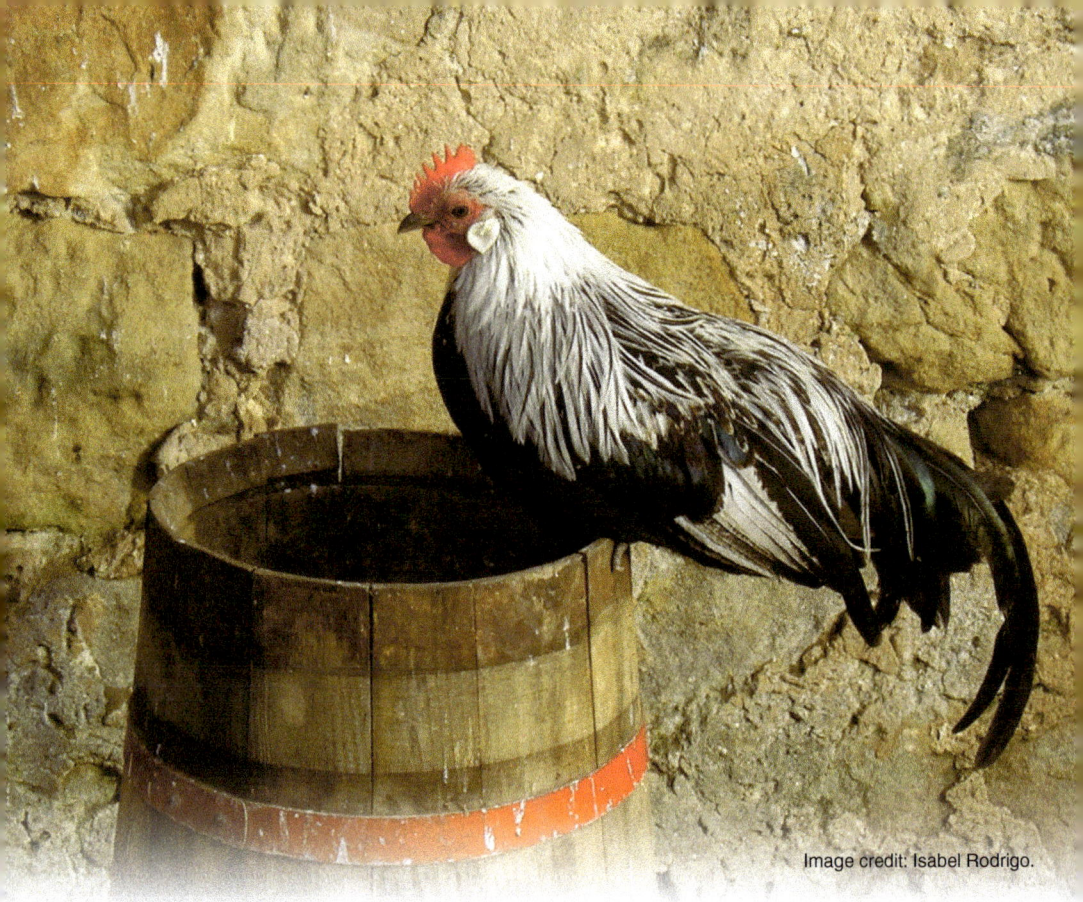
Image credit: Isabel Rodrigo.

and environmental health, collectively, using tools such as surveillance and reporting with an endpoint of improving global health security and achieving gains in development.

(Le Gall *et al.*, 2018)

There is a strong health focus that leaves space for an additional One Welfare definition to complement and expand collaborative approaches.

The concept of One Health aims to deliver added-value benefits rather than just additive benefits to human–animal–environment collaborations. This means that, on top of reducing the risk and improving the health and wellbeing of animals and humans, there are also financial savings and quicker disease detection and response, as well as improved environmental services (Zinsstag *et al.*, 2015).

Following the different approaches to define health, where some restrict it to disease aspects only and others describe it as a holistic state that includes wellbeing (Lerner, 2017), some argue that One Welfare could be an integral part of One Health. However, adopting the wider definition of health under the concept of One Health makes its scope too large when it comes to practical implementation, leaving it to prioritization exercises to decide which aspects of One Health to implement.

Some of the elements included in One Welfare overlap with One Health; yet, by having a separate framework we are able to identify and expose the direct and indirect benefits of animal welfare alone, which are often lost when mixed with animal health topics. Multidisciplinary collaboration groups arranged around One Welfare areas may be different to those with a health focus.

It is also important to ensure that there is a designated and clearly identified body of evidence, including both documented practical examples and scientific analysis, addressing specifically the welfare and wellbeing aspects that often get lost among the disease and public health priorities. While animal welfare issues are acknowledged alongside their connection with human wellbeing and the environment, there is currently not enough research or evidence in the development of combined metrics for human and animal interventions specific to this area. One Welfare creates a framework to enable this, help its recognition and development, and make it happen.

A similar process has taken place on the environmental side, where the Ecohealth concept specifically enables the links between ecosystems, society and health. Here, One Health is an integral part of the Ecohealth concept and the two are complementary and enrich one another (EcoHealth Alliance, 2017).

Some have already reported a need to provide greater importance to animal welfare issues as part of the One Health concept (Wettlaufer *et al.*, 2015). The concept of One Welfare intends to do precisely that.

There needs to be clear rewards and linkages for the human health industry for them to be better engaged. At this point, there is limited evidence to demonstrate the value of collaborative work, and much of the work is anecdotal. Many of the areas covered by One Welfare are not yet fully integrated in medicine handbooks, although some have already been identified as having links with human mental health conditions. Robust evidence has yet to be developed to fully garner the engagement and support needed for a multidisciplinary success at global level. By providing a framework we hope this helps to unify initiatives around the world and make it easier to gather evidence in this area.

Animal and environmental needs are, in many societies, secondary to human needs. But if human health and wellbeing are inextricably linked with animal and environmental health and wellbeing, then they must all be addressed together and their interconnections better understood.

The concept of One Welfare also aims to strengthen the educational aspects behind animal welfare improvements. Emphasizing why different disciplines inherently interact in practice is fundamental (Lerner and Berg, 2015). Interventions need understanding and skill to be successful, but also the right network set-up needs to be in place. For example, help and support may be preferable to prosecution in some on-farm neglect situations, yet this can only be possible if the enforcement authorities are trained and have access to support services that work with them in a collaborative way. There are currently situations where people and animals are not on anyone's radar; however, by setting up multiagency networks and training staff members in a collaborative way of working, there are many opportunities to tackle these aspects in more efficient ways.

Developing multidisciplinary teaching and research goals could be a fundamental tool for changing values and attitudes in different environments. Enhancing educational work and taking into account humans, animals and the environment could awaken different professions to the reality of the new millennium, starting from the premise that sustainability is the basis for any profession.

A unified concept helps to bridge the animal and human sciences and to increase the efficiency of processes (e.g. people of different disciplines being better linked together to increase animal and human welfare simultaneously).

Why a Framework?

One Welfare is a multifaceted concept that captures a broad range of areas. A definition alone does not fully capture the essence of One Welfare. Arranging the different areas within a conceptual framework helps to better understand the multidimensional aspects of the concept. A framework further develops the definition and lays down the multiple considerations connected to the concept, capturing the many aspects of the links between animal welfare, human wellbeing and the environment.

This framework is designed to facilitate collaborative work around and between the different framework sections. The examples and descriptions provided are not full literature reviews of each section, and not necessarily self-limiting, but they have been developed with the intention of providing an indication of areas covered within each section. Being a new framework it will only be natural that, as the concept matures and evolves in society, additional evidence, work programmes, organizations, etc., will develop and hopefully serve in the future as additional good evidence to underpin and help develop further the different framework sections.

Promotion of this framework should enable a wide variety of people to see beyond the interactions and benefits of their own specific remit, looking more broadly at the wider societal considerations and opening up opportunities for developing or improving networks and collaborative set-ups.

One Welfare, One Health and the Benefits of Multidisciplinary and Transdisciplinary Collaboration

In the same way that One Health supports and promotes a truly multi- and interdisciplinary approach (Lerner and Berg, 2015), so does One Welfare. Both the One Health and One Welfare initiatives encourage closer collaboration that can result in benefits in each of the areas they are applied to.

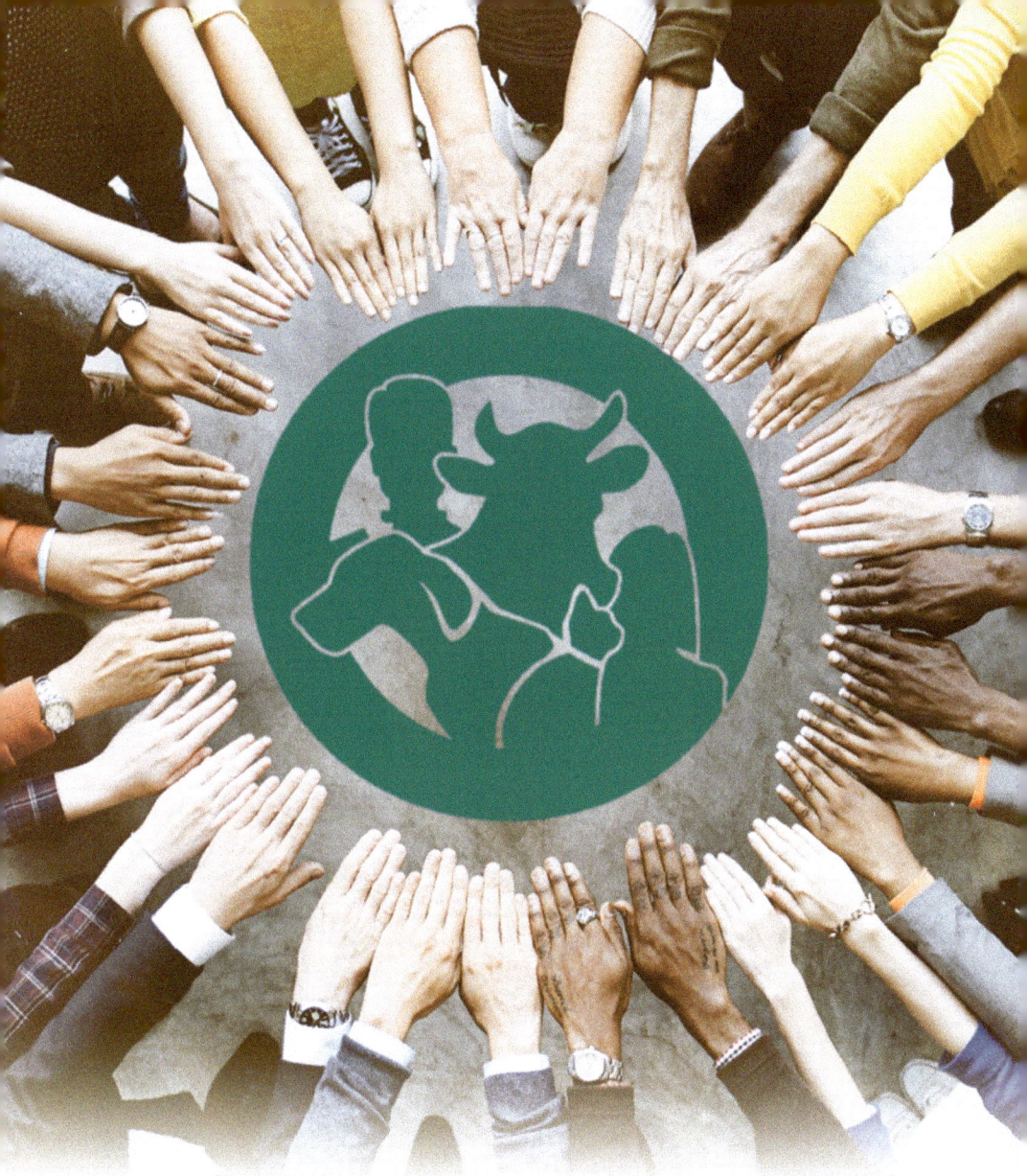

Health is an important part of welfare; improving health always improves welfare, and improving welfare can often result in improvements to health (Broom, 2016). The One Welfare approach can help encourage those who use animals in any way to consider animal welfare as part of their approach and think of them as sentient individuals. This can lead to better treatment and better welfare for all.

The purpose of One Welfare is not to create a parallel structure, separate from One Health, but instead to complement and amplify its benefits within the least developed and known areas of animal, human and environmental

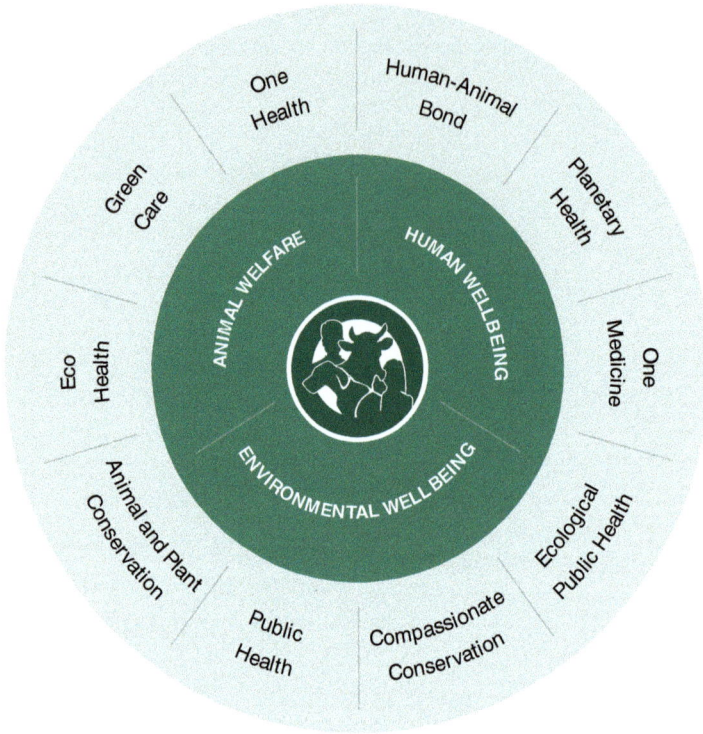

Fig. 1. Interactions of the three key One Welfare elements with other multidisciplinary concepts.

collaborative approaches, with a focus on welfare rather than health. One Welfare serves the role of making explicit the areas of collaboration that have not been developed within One Health or other similar collaborative concepts. It develops a framework in itself to enable the build-up and expansion of an evidence base and practical case study set-up taking into account these areas, which are most times overshadowed by the disease components of One Health.

At a legislative level, improvements setting up the basis to bring closer cooperation between human and animal health and welfare would be beneficial for implementation of a One Health, One Welfare approach (modified from Wettlaufer *et al.*, 2015):

- correlation of human and animal health and welfare explicitly recognized in law;
- regulated cooperation of domestic government departments and institutions for human and animal health, welfare and the environment;
- regulated cooperation with international institutions and governments.

Animal and human data sets are generally focused on disease surveillance; however, there are big gaps when looking in detail at welfare and wellbeing indicators. The deficiency makes it challenging to analyse scientifically correlations between animal welfare, environmental and human wellbeing data. In many cases it can act as a barrier for recognition of existing interconnections, which are often demonstrated anecdotally. Complementing One Health with an explicit welfare component helps to highlight the importance of this element and supports the build-up and expansion of more holistic data sets. This can lead to a better and more robust evidence base that will result in more efficient interventions and better transdisciplinary and interdisciplinary collaboration.

For example, there are established links between ecosystems, poverty and health interactions, and evidence showing that, in developing countries, human sickness is a major cause of falling into and remaining in poverty (Grace, 2016). This is also likely to affect animal welfare, when those humans falling ill have animals under their care and are unable to look after them or provide food. The concept of One Welfare highlights these deeper connections and enables additional tools to help address complex multifactorial scenarios.

The illegal bushmeat trade has been flagged as a threat to both biodiversity and public health under the One Health framework (Chaber, 2016). There are, however, human wellbeing issues connected to illegal activities – and possibly to poverty situations too – as well as animal welfare issues in terms of how bushmeat animals are captured and slaughtered that are often neither exposed nor discussed. Complementing One Health with One Welfare will help to expose and address these types of issues.

In relation to biodiversity and ecosystems, the interrelationship between health and the environment has several angles, such as:

- the influence of biodiversity on disease transmission, where increased biodiversity can have a diluting effect on human transmission of vector-borne and zoonotic disease; however, the chance of introducing super-spreader species might increase the human risk;
- the influence of environmental and landscape homogenization on disease dynamics;
- food security and the impacts of changing biogeochemical cycles on human and system health (Cumming and Cumming, 2015).

To date, the One Health concept has been mainly an approach for health researchers and practitioners at the human, animal and environmental interfaces to work together to mitigate the risks of emerging and re-emerging infectious diseases. This concept was envisaged and implemented as a collaborative global approach to understanding risks for human and animal health (including both domestic animals and wildlife) and ecosystem health as a whole.

While practitioners have focused on implementation of various global standards, the introduction of the concept of One Health has sparked an evidence-based body that goes beyond one discipline. There is, however, a big gap in relation to welfare-focused approaches and we hope that this book helps to enable working methods that better integrate animal welfare.

To achieve a true One Welfare working approach we should aim for coalitions that can deliver cross-training and cross-networks, and which can break down silos to allow for more efficient sharing of information about families in need (adapted from Phillips, 2014).

A more joined-up and multidisciplinary approach could be more efficient and effective. For example, animal welfare indicators can be used as a sign of a farmer (i.e. anyone taking care of livestock on a day-to-day basis, including the farm owner, family and farm staff) being successful or failing to cope and could be used to detect poor farmer health or wellbeing. Equally, poor farmer wellbeing detected by a medical practitioner could indicate a risk of poor animal welfare on the farm. Different professionals could all play a part in improving both farm animal welfare and farmer wellbeing.

While some are of the view that One Welfare is truly under the umbrella of One Health, others believe that One Welfare is broader and encompasses One Health.

We often see the concepts of animal health and animal welfare as separate entities. However, Animal Welfare encompasses five freedoms and domains that include animal health (FAWC, 1993; Mellor, 2016): nutrition, environment, health, behaviour and mental states (Table 1). Based on this basic principle, which is recognized globally, the definition of One Welfare could indeed encompass One Health, instead of complementing it. However, excellent collaborative networks, projects and policies have been built around the concept of One Health, and so the goal is to develop One Welfare as a complement to ongoing One Health programmes, fostering the collaborative approach.

Healthy individuals can suffer poor welfare such as fear, loneliness and boredom. Certain medical treatments (e.g. chemotherapy, many veterinary treatments) can improve health but temporarily harm welfare. At other times poor health occurs without poor welfare (e.g. disabled individuals can be happy and pain free; obesity does not harm welfare in the short term). However, both welfare and health in humans and animals are intimately connected. There is great overlap between the two, as health is a key part of welfare, not something separate.

One Health typically focuses on the health aspects of humans, animals and the environment, and most times is predominantly disease focused. As a result the issues captured under the concept of One Welfare (i.e. psycho–social–economic aspects) are relegated to the periphery. Many agree that welfare is often not included, or is neglected, within the One Health

Table 1. Relationship between One Welfare and the five freedoms, provisions and domains (*adapted from FAWC, 1993 and Mellor, 2016).

Five freedoms, provisions and domain*			One Welfare connections
Nutrition	Freedom from hunger, thirst and malnutrition	Ready access to fresh water and a diet to maintain full health and vigour	Provision of food and water to animals is key to secure their health and welfare, and to underpin human livelihoods
Environment	Freedom from discomfort	Providing a suitable environment including shelter and a comfortable resting area	Environmental resources are connected to both humans and animals Suitable accommodation for animals improves their wellbeing and coexistence with humans
Health	Freedom from pain, injury and disease	Prevention or rapid diagnosis and treatment	Improved animal welfare helps sustain a better immune system and underpin human livelihoods, having positive impacts on productivity, reduction of antimicrobial use or longer working lives Animals sick and/or in pain may display unwanted behaviours which may negatively impact animal–human interactions and compromise welfare
Mental state	Freedom from fear and distress	Ensuring conditions avoid mental suffering	Non-violent handling of animals fosters better human societies and helps prevent human violence and abuse
Behaviour	Freedom to express normal behaviour	Providing sufficient space, proper facilities and company of the animal's own kind	Animals free from behavioural disorders will have better relations with the humans they interact with

approach. Some One Health programmes have recently included welfare; however, this broadens the One Health scope even further. Having a distinct but complementary One Welfare framework provides a space for non-disease-focused disciplines.

One Welfare comprises the behavioural and mental health components of One Health. Similar to the way in which mental health is often neglected in human medicine when compared to infectious disease or acute care, this aspect of One Health runs the risk of being ignored and poorly supported owing to the complexity of the area, and the fact that the evidence is at times still being developed when it relates to animal–human mental states.

To provide sufficient attention to One Welfare issues it is important that the concept develops recognition of its unique reality. To date, One Health focuses very much on physical health, and not all welfare domains have been considered. It could be argued that One Health and One Welfare are different modes of the same concept. In terms of human welfare there is also a great overlap between mental health issues and human–animal welfare which One Health has not fully encompassed. One Welfare helps fill that gap and creates a space for discussion outside of a disease focus.

For One Welfare and One Health to be most effective, a close link is desirable and it would be best if a true One Health–One Welfare approach develops, encompassing all aspects of the broad scope covered. Incorporating a unified approach to One Health and One Welfare is a proposal that aims to break silos and benefit humans, animals and the planet.

Introduction to the One Welfare Framework and Definition

> One Welfare describes the interrelationships between animal welfare, human wellbeing and the physical and social environment.

The concept of One Welfare is a collaborative approach for integrating animal welfare, human wellbeing and the environment, with an end point of improving global welfare and achieving gains in development.

It encompasses multi-, inter- and transdisciplinary ways of working. It is a three-dimensional concept that covers a number of areas and intends to help to integrate animal welfare within other disciplines for a more comprehensive and holistic approach at individual, community and global level. It goes beyond individual welfare and also comprises the wider aspects of societal welfare.

One Welfare can enable networks of public and private stakeholders with the objective to improve global objectives.

The World Health Organization (WHO) defines health as a 'state of complete physical, mental and social wellbeing and not merely the absence of disease or infirmity' (WHO, 2018). In this book welfare and wellbeing are considered equivalent and go beyond the definition of health to comprise emotion and the transient state that is connected to welfare, and the terms 'animal welfare' and 'human wellbeing' mean 'the state when individuals have the psychological, social and physical

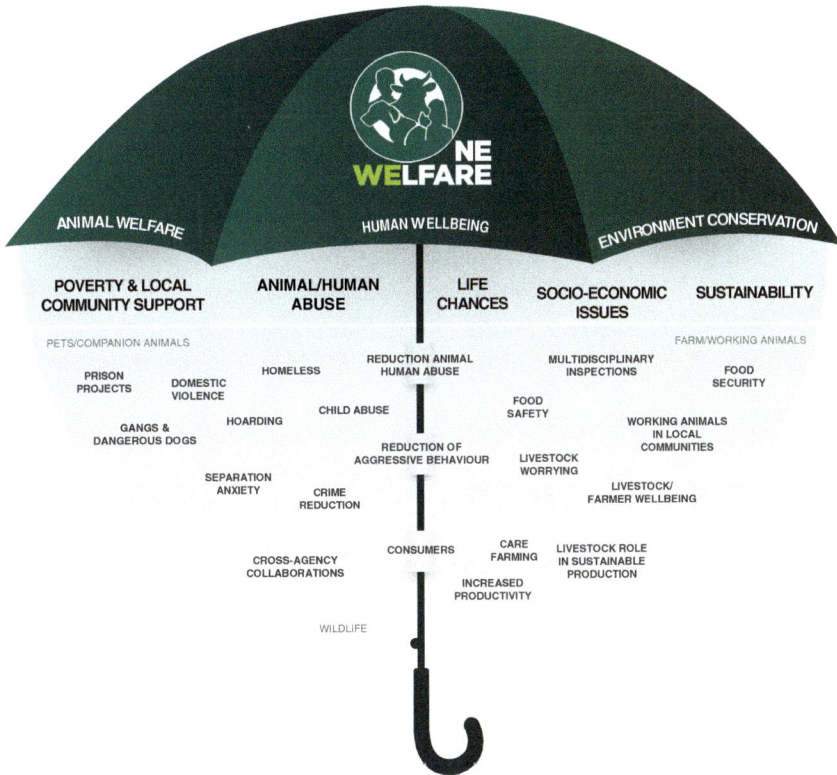

Fig. 2. The One Welfare Umbrella highlights the multiple interconnections between animal welfare, human wellbeing and environmental aspects.

resources they need to meet a particular psychological, social and/or physical challenge' (Dodge *et al.*, 2012).

Overall, health and welfare are inextricably linked and partially overlap when we speak about the term 'quality of life'. 'Health' most often refers to the state of being free from disease, while the terms 'welfare' and 'wellbeing' more often relate to mental and emotional states. Generally you cannot have positive welfare without good health. In a similar way, good welfare will support and be connected to good health.

The 'umbrella approach' is the most important element of the conceptual framework of One Welfare in terms of its multidisciplinary and interdisciplinary perspective oriented to improve collaborative work. These aspects must be considered to develop paths, methods and balances of priorities that can include animal welfare as an integrated (and not peripheral) part of social and environmental concerns.

The interconnections between the three key facets of One Welfare can be multiple and varied. They encompass complex and three-dimensional multifaceted aspects that look at the individual, the community and the global level.

The One Welfare Framework

The One Welfare Framework is made up of five sections, numbered in no particular order of priority. It is as follows:

- Section 1: The connections between animal and human abuse and neglect.
- Section 2: The Social Implications of Improved Animal Welfare.
- Section 3: Animal Health and Welfare, Human Wellbeing, Food Security and Sustainability.
- Section 4: Assisted Interventions Involving Animals, Humans and the Environment.
- Section 5: Sustainability: Connections Between Biodiversity, the Environment, Animal Welfare and Human Wellbeing.

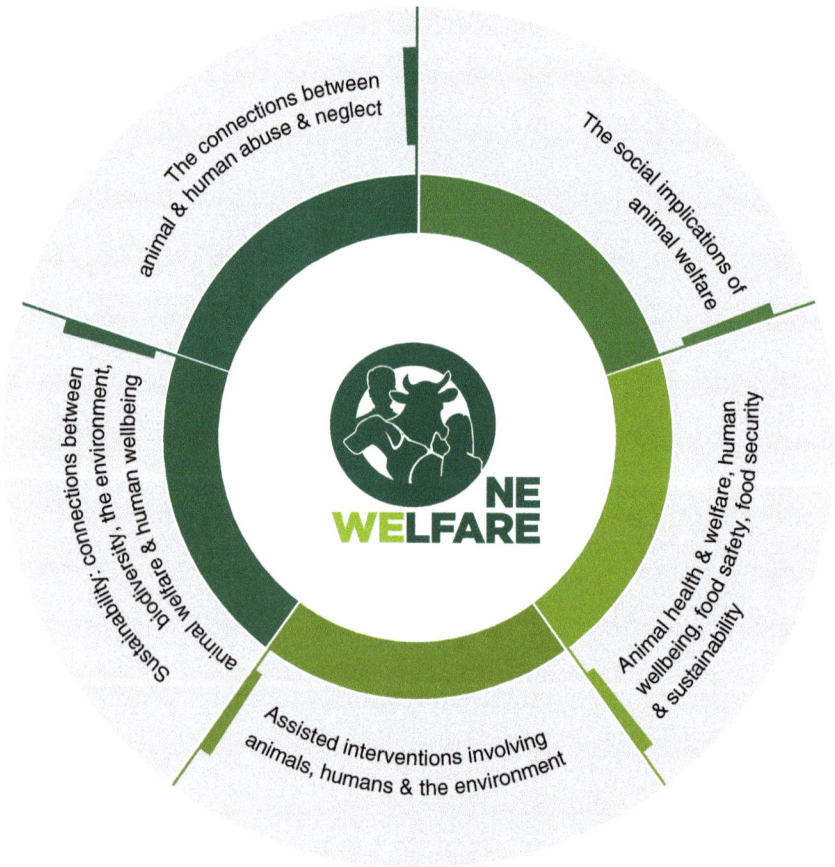

Fig. 3. The One Welfare Framework is made up of five sections.

References

Broom, D.M. (2016) Animal Welfare in the European Union. http://www.europarl. europa.eu/RegData/etudes/STUD/2017/583114/IPOL_STU(2017)583114_EN.pdf (accessed 21 August 2017).

Chaber, A.-L. (2016) Illegal meat trade: a threat to both biodiversity and public health. One Health for the real world: zoonoses, ecosystems and wellbeing. Abstract. https://www.zsl.org/sites/default/files/media/2016-03/One%20Health%20 Abstract%20book_final.pdf (accessed 8 February 2018).

Cumming, D.H.M. and Cumming, G.S. (2015) One Health: An ecological and conservation perspective. In: Zinsstag, J. Schelling, E., Waltner-Toews, D., Whittaker, M. and Tanner, M. (eds) *One Health: The Theory and Practice of Integrated Health Approaches*. CAB International, Wallingford, UK, p. 43.

EcoHealth Alliance (2017) Prevent, prepare and respond: economics of One Health to confront disease threats. Report of workshop 30 January–2 February 2017. https:// www.ecohealthalliance.org/wp-content/uploads/2017/10/Prevent-Prepare-and-Respond-Economics-of-One-Health-to-Confront-Disease-Threats_Workshop-Report.pdf (accessed 7 February 2018).

FAWC (1993) *Second Report on Priorities for Research and Development in Farm Animal Welfare*. Department of Environment, Food and Rural Affairs and Farm Animal Welfare Council (FAWC), London.

Grace, D. (2016) *The Economics of One Health: Ecosystem–Poverty–Health Interactions. One Health for the Real World: Zoonoses, Ecosystems and Wellbeing*. ZSL and The Royal Society, London.

Le Gall, F.G., Plante, C.A., Berthe, F.C.J., Bouley, T., Seifman, R.M., Karesh, W.B. and Machalaba, C.C. (2018) *Operational framework for strengthening human, animal and environmental public health systems at their interface* (English). World Bank Group, Washington, D.C., p. 11. Available at: http://documents. worldbank.org/curated/en/70371517234402168/pdf/WP-P133691-PUBLIC.pdf (accessed 28 February 2018).

Lerner, H. (2017) *Conceptions of Health and Disease in Plants and Animals. Part 2*. In: Schramme, T. and Edwards, S. (eds) *Handbook of the Philosophy of Medicine*. Springer, Dordrecht, Germany, pp. 1–15.

Lerner, H. and Berg, L. (2015) The concept of health in One Health and some practical implications for research and education: what is One Health? *Infection Ecology and Epidemiology* 5, 10.3402/iee.v5.25300.

Mellor, D.J. (2016) Moving beyond the 'Five Freedoms' by updating the 'Five Provisions' and introducing aligned 'animal welfare aims'. *Animals (Basel)* 6(10), 59. https:// www.ncbi.nlm.nih.gov/pmc/articles/PMC5082305/ (accessed 8 February 2018).

Phillips, A. (2014) Understanding the link between violence to animals and people. A guide book for criminal justice professionals. http://www.ndaajustice.org/pdf/ The%20Link%20Monograph-2014.pdf (accessed 8 February 2018).

Wettlaufer, L., Haffner, F. and Zinsstag, J. (2015) The human–animal relationship in the law. In: Zinsstag, J., Schelling, E., Waltner-Toews, D., Whittaker, M. and Tanner, M. (eds) *One Health: The Theory and Practice of Integrated Health Approaches*. CABI, Wallingford, UK, pp. 26–37.

Zinsstag, J., Schelling, E., Waltner-Toews, D., Whittaker, M. and Tanner, M. (eds) (2015) *One Health: The Theory and Practice of Integrated Health Approaches*. CABI, Wallingford, UK.

Section 1

The Connections Between Animal and Human Abuse and Neglect

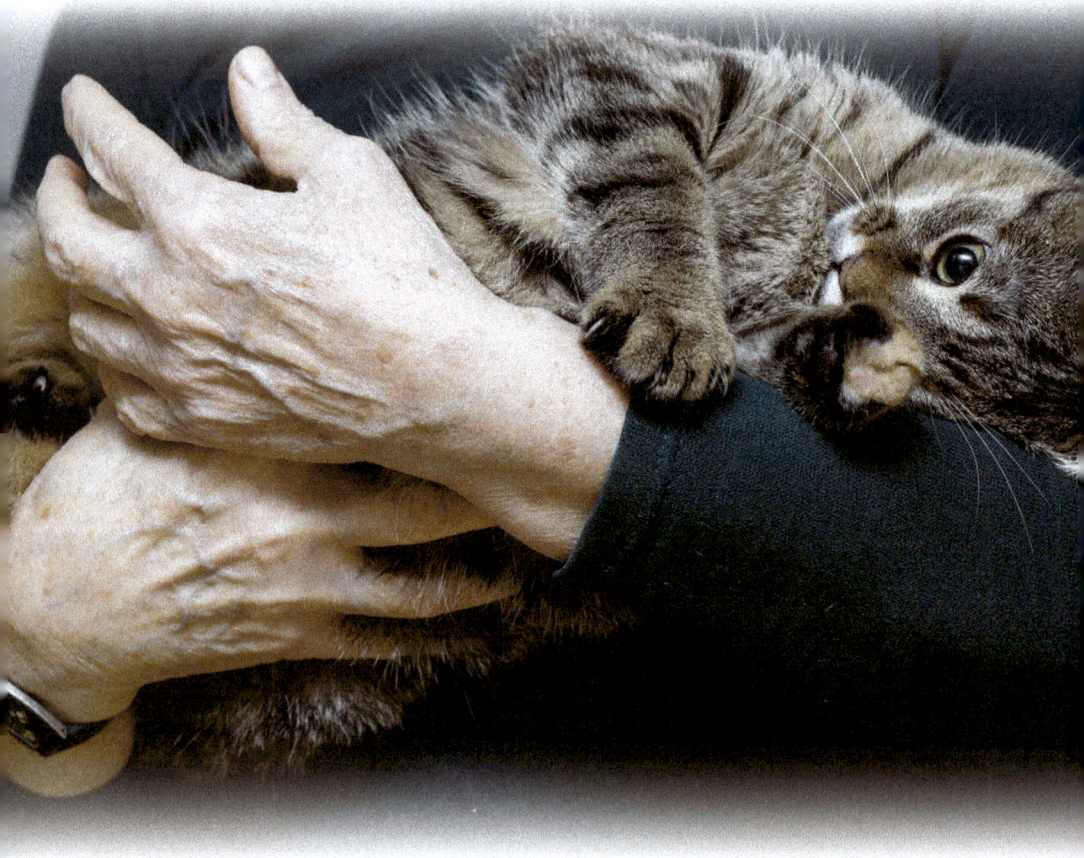

Introduction to Section 1

Section 1 of the One Welfare framework covers all aspects of the links between people and animal interactions where these may result in abuse, neglect or violence. It supports reduction of incidence of crime and violence, in particular domestic violence and maltreatment of vulnerable populations such as elderly people, children and animals, and increases awareness of these issues.

Understanding the links between animal abuse, interpersonal violence (IPV) and neglect can help to identify and therefore possibly prevent abuse or neglect by recognizing low, medium or high risk conditions in various socio-economic environments. Raising awareness that animal abuse and neglect has an influence that goes beyond just the impact on the animal is crucial. Animals presented for non-accidental injury may be indicators of human abuse in a household animal. This can help prevent individual, family and community violence, and may allow early intervention to avert further interpersonal violence.

There is a fundamental difference between neglect (often committed through ignorance) and abuse (deliberate harm of animals to control or coerce another person, or to inflict direct pain on the animal). Abuse towards the vulnerable (human or animal) takes many different forms and generally may be classed as psychological (including controlling or coercive behaviour), physical or sexual assault, or stalking.

Animal abuse offences affect not only the individual animal and immediate family, but can also serve as indicators of deeper social problems at an individual, community or country level. Cultural traditions that inflict pain on, or cause suffering or distress to, animals may also have an indirect impact on people within that population, because these traditions potentially desensitize the community to maltreatment or violence.

Education at all levels of age or experience is a key factor in altering attitudes to animals and vulnerable individuals. If children and adults are taught how to care for animals and, by extension, how to treat them kindly, they acquire social skills including empathy, accountability, responsibility and respect for others. This investment in animal care education may help to reduce both animal abuse and human violence.

Violence, abuse and neglect affecting the vulnerable take many different forms and may be psychological, physical, sexual, social or economic in nature.

Animal abuse does not necessarily mean there is also concurrent human abuse; however, there are compelling studies confirming the connection between animal abuse and neglect, and human abuse and neglect, which include:

- animal abuse as a precursor to, or co-occurring with, other crimes against persons and society;
- animal abuse as an indicator of violence or neglect against vulnerable people within the same household (e.g. when there is animal cruelty or

neglect in a home, there is a likelihood that vulnerable people within the same household, such as children, partners or elderly family members, are being harmed too);
- animal abuse as a mechanism of power and control to harm, intimidate or retaliate against other humans, particularly in cases of IPV, child sexual abuse and elder abuse;
- animal abuse perpetrated by a child may be an indicator that the child has suffered serious neglect or abuse, conduct disorder, oppositional defiant disorder or callousness (psychopathic traits) and may lead to an increased likelihood of other violent behaviours in childhood and adulthood;
- abuse of animals may increase the risk of pet aggression towards adults and children in the same household.

Animal abuse is widely recognized as linking with other types of crime.

> 'If somebody is harming an animal, there is a good chance they also are hurting a human' (National Sheriffs' Association, 2018).

1.1   The Connections between Animal and Human Abuse and Neglect in Practice

Awareness of the link between animal abuse and IPV – as well as with neglect – is increasing globally, and the number of multidisciplinary groups developing projects to intervene in the cycle of violence and neglect cases continues to grow. This section cannot provide a fully comprehensive summary of worldwide initiatives and tools, but it includes basic tools and case studies that are presented to help readers develop collaborative multiagency networks, and to put programmes in place to help human and veterinary healthcare professionals.

Developing One Welfare networks requires the engagement of many stakeholders, including:

- Veterinarians and doctors.
- Animal welfare professionals.
- Animal protection agencies.
- Specialist forensic pathology services.
- Police forces and other relevant law enforcement authorities.
- Local social services representatives (e.g. refuge services, child abuse prevention, adult protective services and social workers).
- Human healthcare and social care professionals (e.g. health visitors, physicians, behavioural health service workers, community nurses and nursery nurses).
- Legal professionals (e.g. prosecutors, judges, and probation and parole officers).
- Academics in diverse fields (e.g. criminology, psychology, sociology).

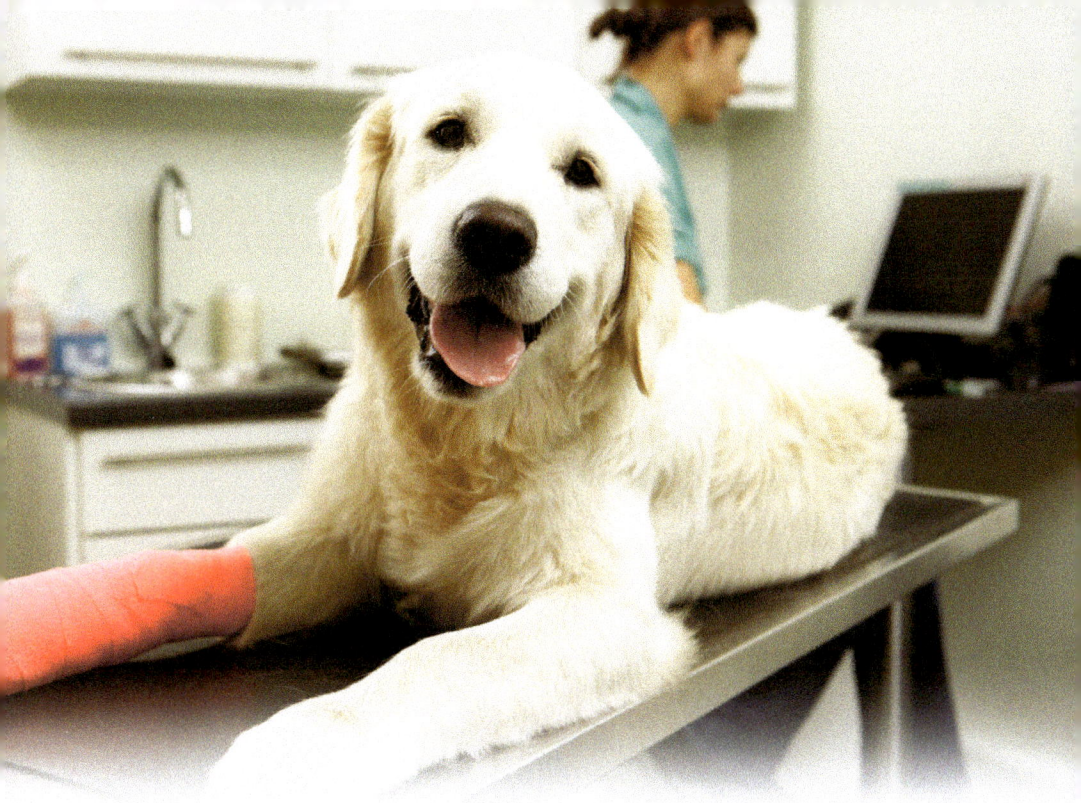

Interventions underpinning this section should provide guidance and supporting documentation for the different professional sectors, containing, as a minimum:

1 Contact details for crisis and advice helplines for:
   - Interpersonal violence.
   - Child protection.
   - Animal protection.
   - Companion animal fostering.
   - Adult protection.
   - Emergency housing services.
2 Information, including:
   - How to recognize abuse and neglect in animals and humans.
   - The role of human and veterinary professionals in recognizing and responding to abuse, neglect or violence cases.
   - Understanding the links from a multidisciplinary, multispecies One Welfare perspective.
   - Enhanced legislation that protects animals and humans.
3 Development of professional codes of practice, legislation and interagency memoranda of understanding for cross-reporting and referrals of cases where multiple manifestations of abuse occur.

Internationally, there is an attitudinal change to inter-personal violence in all its forms. Particularly relevant in the context of this section is increasing intolerance towards violence against women, which is still prevalent in many cultures and countries. Some countries have established 'zero tolerance' policies; for example, Zero Tolerance, the charity established in Scotland to work to prevent violence against women (http://www.zerotolerance.org.uk/). The definition of zero tolerance is 'the act of punishing all criminal or unacceptable behaviour severely, even if it is not very serious' (Cambridge Dictionary: www.dictionary.cambridge.org).

Case Study 1 – VioPet (by Nuria Querol Viñas)

VioPet is a programme coordinated by 'Observatorio de Violencia Hacia los Animales' to raise awareness on the link between animal abuse and family violence and IPV, as well as to help develop foster care programmes for animals of victims who must enter a shelter.

VioPet is part of the 'Sheltering Animals and Families Together' (SAF-T) programme (Allie Phillips, 2011) of the USA. SAF-T is the first programme that guides shelters for victims of violence to house families along with their pets, helping victims to leave their violent homes without leaving their animals behind. This ensures that domestic violence victims who have companion animals do not have to choose between their safety or their companion animal.

VioPet has already been officially supported by four municipalities in Spain, and is also endorsed by several police departments in that country, who may use animal abuse as a red flag for IPV; investigate animal abuse as well as other types of violence; ask the victim if they need special assistance with their companion animal during their stay at a shelter or coordinate with foster homes or humane societies the housing of companion animals.

A pioneer project by 'Ambulorca' (Ambulorca, 2015) that coordinates ambulances for victims of traffic accidents has also endorsed the programme, encouraging for similar arrangements to be made when traffic accidents involve both people and animals. Ambulorca also provides free transportation and foster homes for companion animals of victims of domestic violence.

Case Study 2 – The Links Group (by Freda Scott-Park, The Links Group, UK)

The Links Group is a multiagency group that promotes the welfare and safety of vulnerable children, animals and adults so that they are free from violence and abuse. The main role of the Group is to establish liaisons with other agencies working in the same field with the aim to help all members – humans and animals – of families affected by domestic abuse.

In Great Britain the Links Group offers practical support and advice to vets and human health professionals, through guidance for the veterinary profession in collaboration with the Royal College of Veterinary Surgeons, the British Veterinary Association and the Animal Welfare Foundation. Education is available for members of the veterinary team through the Links Veterinary Training Initiative and by visits to veterinary schools to train undergraduates. An online course in basic animal welfare has been produced to aid human healthcare professionals unfamiliar with animals, who are entering violent households, to evaluate the wellbeing of the pet.

Case Study 3 – The National Link Coalition (by Phil Arkow, National Link Coalition, USA)

The National Link Coalition was formed in 2008 as an independent collaboration among law enforcement, prosecution, child abuse, domestic violence, animal welfare, elder abuse, and veterinary and human healthcare organizations. Its mission is to promote and disseminate research, public policy, programming and public awareness of how animal abuse is linked with other forms of family and community violence. Based in the USA, it has a global outreach of over 3500 participants in 55 nations.

The National Link Coalition believes that multidisciplinary approaches lead to more effective prevention, protection and prosecution of family and community violence. The Coalition's activities include:

- Management of the National Resource Center on The Link Between Animal Abuse and Human Violence (www.nationallinkcoalition.org), which includes the publication of a free monthly newsletter, *The LINK-Letter*, disseminated at global level.
- Initiating and sustaining local and regional community anti-violence coalitions in the USA and 13 other nations, providing a toolkit to help stimulate such task forces.
- Monitoring legislation, including domestic violence protection.
- Protection from abuse orders that include animals; cross-reporting protocols among child abuse, elder abuse and animal cruelty enforcement agencies; animal sexual abuse and hoarding issues; psychological evaluations of animal cruelty offenders; and animal abuse linked with other crimes.
- Maintaining an online bibliography of over 1200 academic citations researching the intersections of child maltreatment, animal abuse, domestic violence, elder abuse, bullying, animal hoarding and animal sexual abuse.
- Conducting multidisciplinary training for professionals. Between 2014 and 2016 the team presented at 320 conferences and 36 webinars in the USA and overseas.
- Publishing materials to aid professionals in the prevention, recognition and response to all forms of family violence.
- Assisting domestic violence organizations to initiate pet support services that enable the entire family to leave abusive situations.
- Maintaining the first national directory of over 6000 community agencies in the USA that investigate allegations of animal, child, elder and domestic abuse.

The National Link Coalition works on the principle that the prevention of family and community violence can best be achieved through species-spanning partnerships. Through the recognition and integration of this understanding into policies and practices, humans and animals will be measurably safer.

Under the One Welfare umbrella, and to capitalize on the global enthusiasm for breaking the cycle of domestic violence, the development of internationally agreed welfare metrics for both animals and humans would be invaluable. The value of the animal as a sentinel of wider abuse within the household should continue to be highlighted in all communications involving domestic abuse.

Medical doctors should be made aware that the human–animal bond (HAB) may provide a useful opportunity to improve the patient–doctor communication axis, leading to better assessments of health, social context and environmental history (Hodgson *et al.*, 2017).

References and Resources

Allie Phillips (2011) About SAF-T. Available at: http://alliephillips.com/saf-tprogram/about-saf-t/ (accessed 26 April 2018).

Ambulorca (2015) AMAR. Available at: http://ambulorca.com/responsabilidad-social/amar (accessed 16 February 2018).

Dodge, R., Daly, A.P., Huyton, J. and Sanders, L.D. (2012) The challenge of defining wellbeing. *International Journal of Wellbeing* 2(3), 222–235. doi:10.5502/ijw. v2i3.4. Available at: https://www.bitc.org.uk/sites/default/files/the_challenge_of_defining_wellbeing_-_dodge_et_al_2012.pdf (accessed 16 February 2018).

Animal Therapy (2018) LINK Bibliography: Bibliography of the Link Between Animal Abuse, Domestic Violence, Child Abuse and Elder Abuse. Available at: http://animaltherapy.net/animal-abuse-human-violence/link-bibliography/ (accessed 14 October 2017).

Hodgson *et al.* (2017) Asking About Pets Enhances Patient Communication and Care: A Pilot Study. *INQUIRY: The Journal of Health Care Organization, Provision, and Financing.* 54, 1–6. Available at: http://journals.sagepub.com/doi/pdf/10.1177/0046958017734030 (accessed 3 May 2018).

HSUS (2008) *First Strike: The Violence Connection*. HSUS, Washington, DC. Available at: http://www.humanesociety.org/assets/pdfs/abuse/first_strike.pdf (accessed 14 October 2017).

National Sheriffs' Association (2018) National Law Enforcement Center on Animal Abuse. Available at: https://www.sheriffs.org/programs/national-law-enforcement-center-animal-abuse (accessed 8 February 2018).

The Links Group (2018) Welcome to The Links Group. Available at: http://www.thelinksgroup.org.uk/ (accessed 14 October 2017).

The National Link Coalition (2018) Resource Materials. Available at: http://nationallinkcoalition.org/resources/articles-research (accessed 14 October 2017).

Phillips, A. (2014) *Understanding the Link Between Violence to Animals and People: a Guidebook for Criminal Justice Professionals*. National District Attorneys Association, Alexandria, Virginia. Available at: http://www.ndaajustice.org/pdf/The%20Link%20Monograph-2014.pdf (accessed 14 October 2017).

NSPCC (n.d.) Understanding the Links: Child Abuse, Animal Abuse and Domestic Violence. NSPCC, London, UK. https://www.nspcc.org.uk/globalassets/documents/research-reports/understanding-links-child-abuse-animal-abuse-domestic-violence.pdf (accessed 14 October 2017).

VioPet (2018) VIOPET: Protegiendo a todas las víctimas de violencia. Available at: http://viopet.org/ (accessed 14 October 2017).

WHO (2018) Constitution of WHO: principles. Available at: http://www.who.int/about/mission/en/ (accessed 8 February 2018).

Section 2

The Social Implications of Improved Animal Welfare

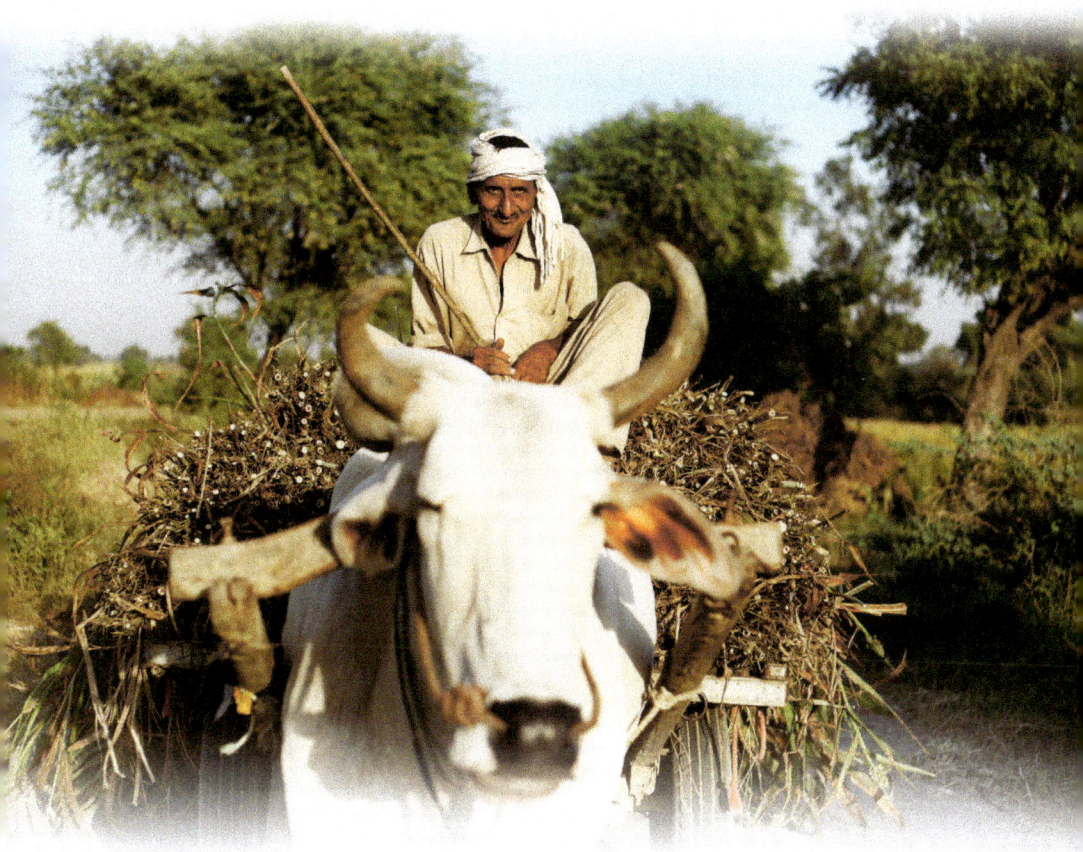

Section 2 of the One Welfare framework covers the connection between poor states of human and animal welfare. It examines cases involving animal welfare, socio-economic indicators and offences in different social contexts, including those taking place within underprivileged communities. Improvements in animal welfare can support interventions tackling social issues (such as homelessness, hoarding, dog fighting and separation anxiety). Integrating animal welfare as part of general livelihood improvement programmes, including disaster and war responses, is seen as key to success.

We all live in a social configuration in which we have a shared life between humans and other animals. Animal and human welfare are interlinked in socio-economic issues, and poor animal welfare can generally be used as an indicator of much wider human wellbeing. We interact with animals in different ways within rural, urban or working environments. Underprivileged communities may be found in inner-city, suburban, rural and remote locations, and in any situations where resources – such as sources of finance or education – are limited.

This section focuses on the interactions at both individual and community levels and has been divided into a number of subsections to help in highlighting the multiple angles within which animal welfare is linked to human wellbeing within a social context. The section does not intend to provide a fully comprehensive list of interactions, but to include sufficient examples to enable readers to develop and implement initiatives within their own localities.

Overall, this section relates to areas where improved animal welfare goes beyond animal protection to reach human support.

2.1   Companion Animal Welfare

Companion animals are likely to be the ones interacting most closely with humans. They are part of the daily lives of many and, in most circumstances, they share housing and have become one more member of the family.

The welfare of companion animals is intertwined with that of those who share their lives with them. Compromising their welfare, whether intentionally or not will inevitably affect the family and – depending on the actual issue – also affect others such as neighbours or people or other animals who interact with the family or the companion animal itself.

Behavioural problems reported by the owners of companion animals can adversely affect the human–animal bond (HAB) and can impact directly on the owner and their family, but may also have negative effects on the wider community. The behaviours involved may be the result of inappropriate learning or lack of training and these can often be addressed by training interventions. However, many companion animal behaviours which are reported by owners or by communities as being problematic are the outward manifestation of an emotional health issue for the animal. Such emotional disturbances can be reactive and result from suboptimal environments, which do not meet the species-specific environmental needs of the animal. Others are the result of compromised emotional health related to abnormalities of neurotransmitter function (Sarah Heath, pers. comm., 2017). The involvement of veterinary specialists in behavioural medicine can address not only the emotional health issue of the companion animal, but also highlight the negative effects on human health and welfare. Collaboration with human health professionals may be needed in some cases, but the opportunity for owners and their families to discuss the situation in detail can be therapeutic in itself (Sarah Heath, pers. comm., 2017). It is important for the issue of non-human animal emotional health to be given equal consideration to their physical health, and for veterinary intervention in behavioural cases to be undertaken using a One Welfare approach.

Education becomes a key component where welfare problems may arise as a result of non-intentional abuse through miscommunication and misunderstanding which stems from human lack of understanding of the other species they live with. This may materialize as ignorance, neglect or abuse when, in fact, the actual root cause is a lack of basic care knowledge.

Separation-related behaviours

When animals are left alone for prolonged periods some may suffer from separation-related behaviours or related behavioural problems which can

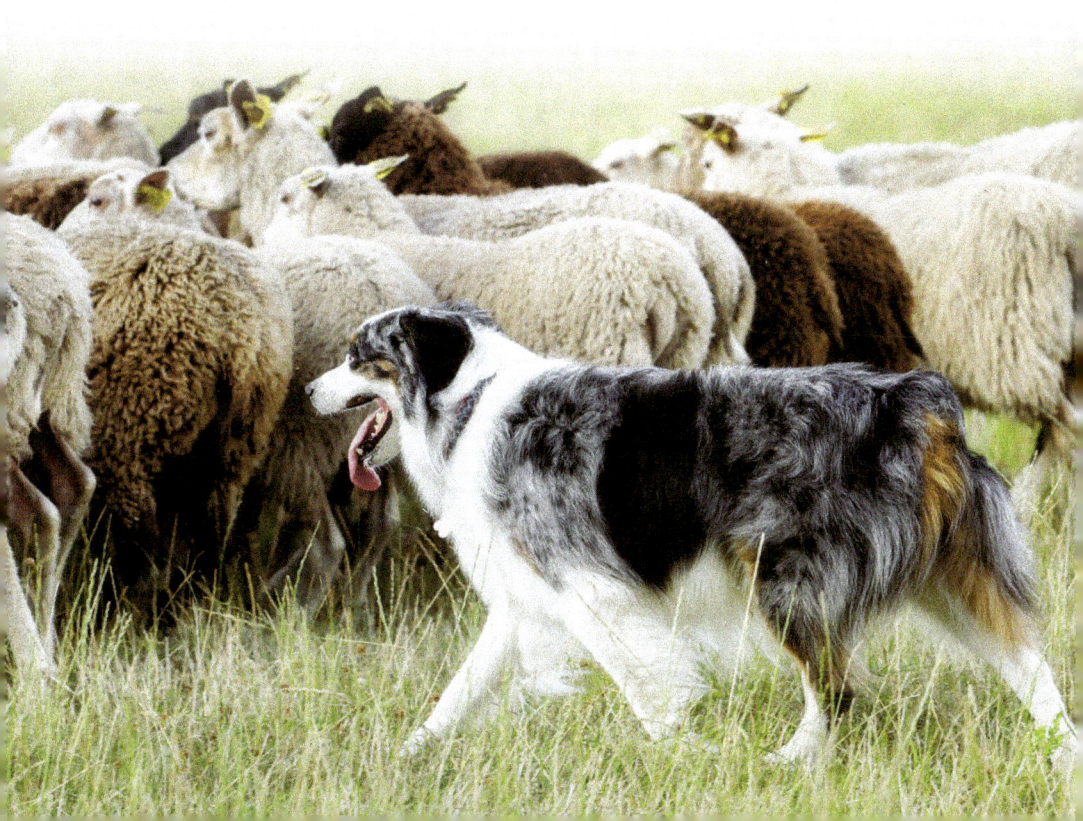

have a range of emotional motivations. The behavioural outcomes of those motivations can be similar, and reports of howling, barking, destruction or toileting in the owner's absence are common. While the impact on the owner may be the first consideration, it is important to remember that these behaviours can also impact on the immediate family, the direct neighbours and even the wider community. The welfare impact can be significant for both the human and non-human animals involved. Other and more subtle behavioural outcomes, such as pacing, restlessness or repetitive behaviours may primarily affect the companion animal and are at risk of being considered less important because of their reduced impact on humans.

Interventions such as raising awareness of pet owners and rearing companion animals appropriately so that they can integrate into domestic life can help prevent these welfare issues. Introducing socialization at early stages under the supervision of a trained animal behaviourist can support efforts to help prevent these welfare issues. Understanding emotional health in companion animals and the importance of maximizing emotional resilience and stability is the key, alongside increased education about species-specific environmental needs and the requirement for environmental optimization (Sarah Heath, pers. comm., 2017). Genetic selection may also have an influence on these aspects, and has not yet been fully explored.

Case Study 4 – Separation-related distress (by Sarah Heath, England)

When Rosie came home from work to find a handwritten note from her neighbour on the door mat she did not initially comprehend the ramifications. The note informed Rosie that her pet dog Harry had been howling and barking for hours while she had been at work, and that the neighbour had been talking to other neighbours about what action they should take.

At that moment Rosie experienced a mixture of reactions including concern for Harry and sadness at the thought of him being distressed, guilt at having to leave him alone for so long while she was working, and worry about the effect on her relationship with her neighbours and the potential action that they might take.

When a letter from the environmental health department of her local council arrived just 3 days later an additional response – anger – began to take hold. How could her neighbours have reported her without giving her a chance to sort things out? How could they be so lacking in empathy and understanding?

Rosie lived alone and after being unemployed for a long time she had managed to secure employment in a supermarket. She only worked for 4 hours a day but the supermarket was a long way from her home and she did not drive. Taking public transport meant that the journey to and from work was long and could often be extended due to the unreliability of the buses on that route. Without any family nearby Rosie felt that she had no choice but to leave Harry home alone for 6–7 hours a day.

This case highlights the role of a One Welfare approach. Harry's howling was not only indicative of his own emotional distress, but also highlighted difficulties

Continued

> **Case Study 4.** Continued.
>
> within Rosie's personal situation and their impact on her wellbeing, and also the impact of Harry's behaviour on relationships within the local community.
>
> Changing Harry's emotional response to his owner's absence will take time and in the meantime Rosie does not have the financial capacity to take advantage of pet sitting or dog walking services, which may have been beneficial.
>
> Talking to her neighbours face to face and explaining that she was getting professional help to deal with Harry's behaviour helped to improve understanding and empathy. It also opened up conversations which had practical benefits, such as finding out that one of her neighbours who was retired and at home all day had recently been bereaved, and would relish the opportunity to have Harry for company while Rosie was at work.
>
> The community's perception of Harry changed overnight – rather than being seen as the annoying howling dog he became seen as a canine social worker. Rosie became integrated into her community and found social support which made an enormous difference to her life. Harry was given the social interaction he needed to change his expectations and alter his emotional response to spending shorter periods of time at home alone while Rosie worked.

Responsible dog ownership

Caring for animals can contribute to creating a sense of responsibility, which helps people overcoming social issues. There are positive impacts on people from owning or caring for a pet and nowadays there are increasing examples and projects supporting pet ownership in different ways. However, it is important to note that not everyone is able to care for pets properly and not every pet might be suitable for a given individual. This may be due to a number of reasons, including the physical space where they live, their mental health condition or the education and knowledge they have about the pet they intend to keep.

There is a direct benefit from using cases of improvements in animal welfare to aid social intervention. For example, hospital admissions for bites and strikes by dogs amongst people living in the most deprived areas of England are reported to be three times as high as in the least deprived areas (NHS, 2014). By improving responsible dog ownership there could be a positive impact both on the welfare of dogs, owners and those affected by the bites or strikes.

Community dog programmes are now widespread across the world to encourage responsible dog ownership. Some of these are already linked to social service providers, such as housing, or animal infectious disease control programmes, such as rabies control. It would be helpful to help disseminate best practice examples of these collaborative approaches although they are not generally well documented in a systematic, evidence-based format. It would also help to build up tools to effectively and systematically

monitor these types of interventions, such as, for example, correlations between the Human Development Indexes in different societies and animal
welfare status in different scenarios within each society.

In rural areas, interventions that educate owners on responsible dog
ownership and dog control can help prevent dog attacks to livestock. The
impact of this extends to livestock welfare and that of the farming community, which can be affected by financial losses, distress and additional negative factors such as depression (NSA, 2016).

Case Study 5 – National Sheep Association Annual Survey (UK) (by Nicola Smith, National Sheep Association, UK)

Following a series of serious incidents where dogs out of control in livestock
fields caused deaths and farm losses, the National Sheep Association in the UK
(NSA) has been involved in numerous efforts to reduce these incidents. For example, a number of case studies showing the impact on sheep flocks and sheep
farmers of dogs out of control has been collated and is publically available on its
website. The NSA has also developed materials to help address the issue and
raise public awareness, including a 'sheepwise' campaign aimed at dog owners.
This displays a short film featuring first-hand accounts of the devastation caused
when dogs worry sheep, covering both the anguish that dog owners face, along
with a potential criminal prosecution if they fail to control their dogs properly in
the countryside. It also stresses the negative impact on farmers and sheep welfare by describing the devastation of seeing lambs or ewes attacked and killed
by dogs.

As part of this work the NSA created a nationwide survey that demonstrates the
consequences of these attacks for:

• The livestock: number of dead, escapes, abortions, injury or euthanasia
  incidents.
• The farmer: stress, financial losses, depression, etc.
• The dog: shot on site or court-ordered euthanasia.
• The owner: financial payments through compensation, emotional stress from
  loss of dog.

Finally, resources to address this welfare problem in the farming community
and dog ownership sector have focused on educational campaigns by providing
posters and signs for the public, advice to farmers and raising awareness among
police forces of the importance of treating this crime seriously.

Animal hoarding

Animal hoarding involves one or more individuals who gather animals beyond the typical number of pets. This number will vary depending on the environment, care provision facilities, space, etc. As a result they fail to provide
minimum care standards and may not be able to understand their failure

Table 2.1. Animal hoarding disorder signs.

Persistent difficulty in parting from kept animals and possessions
Cluttered living spaces
Poor health and welfare of the hoarder and kept animals
Environmental nuisance such as accumulation of litter, bad smells or noise.
Excessive acquisition of animals (at times also items) that they are not able to care
   for, do not need or for which no space or facilities are available
Limited insight into their difficulties and reluctant to seek help
Evidence of unlawful activities

Adapted from DSM-5 (2013) and Mataix-Cols (2014). Not all signs may be present
in each case.

to recognize the effects on animal welfare, human family members and the surrounding environment (Patronek *et al.*, 2006). This can be linked to a human need to accumulate animals and control them, and most times supersedes the needs of the animals or people involved. The need to accumulate items has been described as 'hoarding disorder', a mental health condition where an individual has persistent difficulty in discarding or parting with possessions, alongside other defined signs (DSM-5, 2013). Hoarding can affect the living environment and, in severe cases, put individuals and their kept animals at risk of fire, poor sanitation and other health and welfare risks. Further clinical trials have been recommended to ascertain whether animal hoarding is a special manifestation of the 'hoarding disorder' or whether it is instead linked to other mental health problems (Mataix-Cols, 2014).

Table 2.1 is a summary of possible signs that might be identified in cases of animal hoarding.

Animal hoarding is a One Welfare issue because it affects animal welfare as well as the wellbeing of the hoarders, their families and the community around them. It can also be associated with a number of neurological and psychiatric conditions (Pertusa *et al.*, 2010), which may also be connected to elder abuse, child abuse and self-neglect, as well as costs to local government and support organizations.

Three types of animal hoarder have been described (Table 2.2), with some hoarding displaying signs of a combination of categories:

- The overwhelmed caregiver, who initially provides adequate care but is then unable to cope; they generally understand that a problem has gradually developed though they may minimize it. The cause may be social isolation or a change in their circumstances; in most cases they are happy to accept assistance and support.
- The rescue hoarder, whose main intention is to save animals from euthanasia at any expense; the cause is rooted in the belief that they are

Table 2.2. Animal hoarder characteristics (adapted from Patronek et al., 2006).

Overwhelmed caregiver	Rescuer hoarder	Exploiter hoarder
Exhibits some awareness of problems with animal care, more reality-based than other types of hoarder	Has strong sense of mission to save animals, which leads to unavoidable compulsion	Tends to have sociopathic characteristics or personality disorder
Acquires animals passively and finds problem triggered by a change in circumstances or resources – social, economic or medical, e.g. loss of spouse who helped care for animals, onset of illness or disability, loss of job or income	Acquires animals actively rather than passively and believes they are the only one who can provide adequate care	Acquires animals actively rather than passively, purely to serve own needs
Makes an initial effort to provide proper care, but eventually gets overwhelmed, and is unable to solve problems effectively	Starts with adequate resources for animal care but finds it hard to refuse requests to take more animals. Numbers of animals gradually overwhelm capacity to provide minimal care	Believes their knowledge is superior to that of all other people; adopts the role of expert with extreme need to control
Has a strong attachment to animals as family members and finds attachment to animals a bigger issue than control Tends to minimize rather than deny the problems	The initial rescue-followed-by-adoption pattern is replaced by rescue-only care Fears death (of animals and self) and opposes euthanasia	Lacks empathy for people or animals; indifferent to the harm caused to animals or people Tends toward extreme denial of the situation
Tends to be withdrawn and isolated, possibly due to physical infirmity, with self-esteem linked to role as a caregiver. Needs guardianship in many cases	Is not necessarily socially isolated; may work with an extensive network of enablers and be more engaged in society, therefore less amenable to intervention via social services	Has superficial charm and charisma – very articulate, skilled in crafting excuses and explanations, and capable of presenting an appearance that conveys believability and competence to officials, the public and the media. Is manipulative and cunning, self-concerned and narcissistic. Lacks guilt, remorse or social conscience

Continued

Table 2.2. Continued.

Overwhelmed caregiver	Rescuer hoarder	Exploiter hoarder
Has more tendency towards some psychological disorders, including mental health conditions such as mood disorders, schizoaffective disorders or psychotic disorders		Demonstrates predatory behaviour – will lie, cheat or steal without remorse and potentially has a plan to use these tools to achieve own ends
Allows intervener to gain entry, client more likely to respect the system and comply with recommendations; is less deliberately secretive	Avoids authorities or impedes their access	Plans to evade the law and beat the system, such as dispersing animals to other animal hoarders or friends
Has fewer issues with authorities or need to control animals or property		Rejects authority or any outsider's legitimate concern over animal care

the only ones who can adequately care for the animals, and they have issues declining to care for additional animals to care for. They may work alone or in a network but generally avoid authorities.

- The exploiter hoarder, who mainly looks for self-benefit. The causes for this are complex and are linked to characters who may come across as charming, articulate, manipulative and cunning. They may also be self-concerned and do not express remorse or guilt, evading the law and lying, cheating or stealing if necessary (Patronek *et al.*, 2006). This may occur in conjunction with other unlawful activities, such as financial crime (Sylvester and Baranyk, 2011a,b).

A multidisciplinary approach to address animal hoarding should include those related to community health and welfare, such as those looking after animal welfare, human health and mental health, housing, law enforcement, sanitation and the environment (Patronek *et al.*, 2006). Interventions such as animal euthanasia, rehoming, human therapy, social support or enforcement are examples of actions that may be taken to address hoarding situations. However, the ideal solution for each particular case needs to be carefully studied and tailored to the individual circumstances and resources available. The welfare of first responders is also a key element that needs to be accounted for, with provision of adequate support to them too.

Case Study 6 – Prairie Mountain Inter-Agency Hoarding Coalition (by PMIHC) (PMIHC, Canada)

The Prairie Mountain Inter-Agency Hoarding Coalition (PMIHC) is a multi-agency group in the western part of Manitoba, Canada. The group came together in 2010 to tackle issues of hoarding and domestic squalor (H+DS) in the region. The PMIHC was founded by a multidisciplinary group consisting of: public health inspectors,[1] fire inspectors and animal welfare veterinarians. Each discipline shared common concerns about the growing numbers of complex H+DS cases trending in the area.

In essence, these responders noticed that they were unwittingly addressing the same calls with very little interagency coordination or common understanding of each other's mandates and legislative constraints. Before long, these officials realized that they singularly lacked the tools and resources necessary to achieve positive outcomes. It was also obvious to each group that mental health disorders were an underlying issue for each H+DS case and that, to be successful, a more interprofessional approach was needed.

From its inception, the concept of 'One Welfare' was also core to efforts. The following case summaries highlight some of the ways in which the PMIHC has progressed with respect to response, recovery and prevention strategies:

Case 1: 'Level 5' hoarding and entry warrants

A landlord who owned over a dozen rental properties kept them in varying degrees of dilapidation, rapidly becoming unsuitable for tenants to occupy. The owner compulsively collected household items, furniture, rubbish, clothing, etc., and completely filled up four dwellings with contents. There were between two to three cats per dwelling, suffering neglect and forced to live in squalor, their primary purpose being to control mice and rats.

The individual cut out cavities in the walls and purchased intermodal shipping containers to 'store treasures'. Neighbours complained to local authorities about the fire and health hazards on these properties. The owner was a charming individual with excellent cognitive skills, but was very evasive despite her friendly demeanour. She consistently refused entry to regulators and invoked her rights of privacy. In the end, health officials had to collect evidence and witness statements to obtain 'entry warrants'.

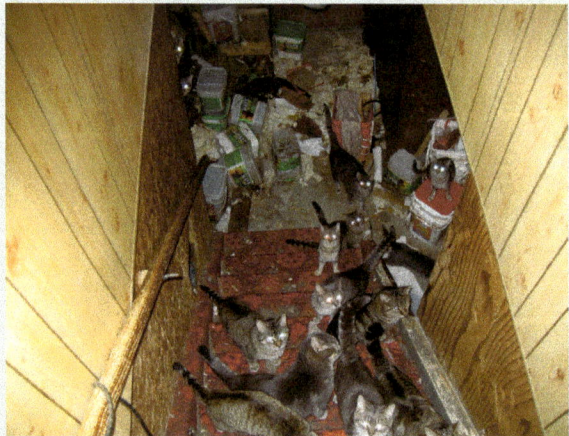

Continued

> **Case Study 6.** Continued.
>
> Outcome: The individual did manage to comply and sell off her properties, but only after being compelled to do so by regulatory orders. This case illustrated the need for a tool to measure the severity of hoarding to put things into context. The Institute for Challenging Disorganization had previously developed an intuitive and user-friendly 'Clutter-Hoarding Scale™ (ICD, 2016) that PMIHC was able to adopt and use in its routine operations.
>
> **Case 2: Cat hoarding, toxic ammonia levels and first responders**
>
> An ageing couple struggling with health issues and loneliness due to an 'empty nest' allowed their domestic cat population to surge to over 25 animals. Conditions in the home deteriorated such that the squalor created ammonia levels in excess of ten times the safe chronic exposure levels. (AISDR, 2004) A coordinated response was mounted involving officials from fire, environmental health, animal welfare, mental health, police and ambulance services.
>
> Outcome: The couple was successfully relocated and connected with appropriate services and referrals. The animals were seized and put into care, but many were euthanized due to health complications. This case illustrated the need for ensuring that air quality assessments are part of ensuring both occupant and responder safety. It also underlined the fact that first responders[2] are core to early detection and there is a need for awareness and upstream coordination. A 'First Responders Guide' and an 'Initial Intake/Assessment Form[3] was created to further improve coalition efforts.
>
> [1] Also referred to as Environmental Health Officers in various countries.
> [2] Ambulatory personnel indicated that they had been aware of the situation for 4–5 years, but were not aware of how to report to an appropriate authority.
> [3] Copies of both documents are available upon request by emailing the PMHIC Secretariat (For details, visit: http://prairiemountainhealth.ca/index.php/9-programs-services/36-healthy-communities)

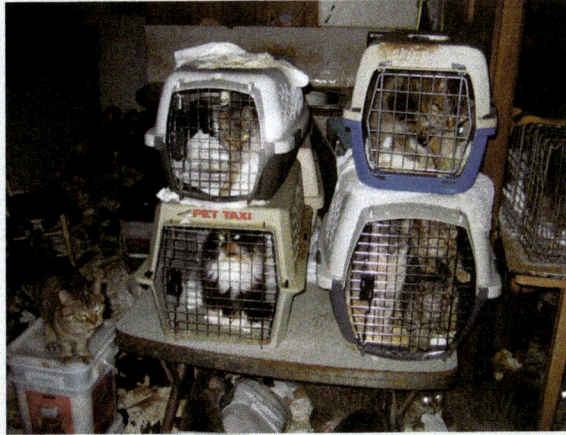

Loneliness, homelessness, ageing and interrelations with companion animals

While not often discussed, the role of companion animals in urban communities can be key to individual livelihoods. They provide support, with a number of psychosocial benefits such as decreased depression, decreased anxiety, decreased loneliness, improved morale or increased social inter-action (pets as catalysts) (Johnson, 2009).

These animals will generally have a role at the local community support level, and support efforts to help address physical, psychological and social support (Scanlon, 2016).

Social care, mental health and public health services will care for the human wellbeing aspects and it is increasingly recognized that animals are important as part of this. Enabling frameworks that link these professionals with animal welfare experts can help in their task of taking a more compre-hensive approach.

Case Study 7 – Our Special Friends (by Belinda Johnston, Our Special Friends, England)

Our Special Friends (OSF) – 'helping people and animals help each other' – is a veterinary-led charity based in Suffolk, UK. Its work is focused on the local com-munity to help isolated and vulnerable people, of any age, to continue to benefit from the companionship of animals through financial need, physical disability or ill health, enhancing wellbeing through practical and emotional support services and animal-assisted activities.

Its free support is provided by local volunteers, and by working in collaboration with human health and social care organizations, as well as with veterinarians

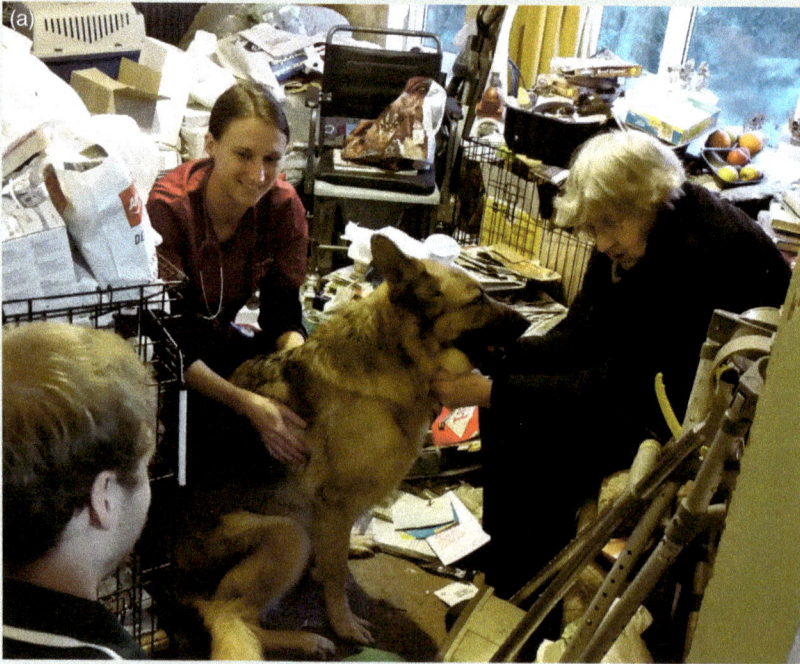

Continued

Case Study 7. Continued.

and animal welfare charities. By encouraging local residents to volunteer, it also helps create community cohesion and mutually beneficial empowering relationships.

Reaching people through their love of animals enables OSF to act as a high-impact, low-cost, early-intervention health and welfare initiative for both humans and animals. OSF bridges the gap between existing services, filling the void with a collaborative multidisciplinary approach. By targeting socially isolated cases OSF often identifies unmet health and social care needs, which may be concealed from others, and helps link those in need to other social and health care providers.

OSF provides support at three key levels:

- Practical:
  help with dog walking or cleaning the cat tray;
  enabling a pet to stay with its owner;
  sourcing, introducing and monitoring a new pet;
  regular visits from a 'visiting' dog and volunteer.

- Emotional:
  coping with difficult pet decisions;
  pet bereavement and the impact of loss;
  pet care planning to give peace of mind and avoid crises.

- Organizational:
  work with veterinarians, hospices and other organizations;
  ○ referral to specialists when support is needed.

Two brief examples of work undertaken by OSF follow.

A woman in her mid-70s had relied on her dog, Poppy, while caring for her late husband (image a). Soon after his death, she too was diagnosed with a terminal illness.

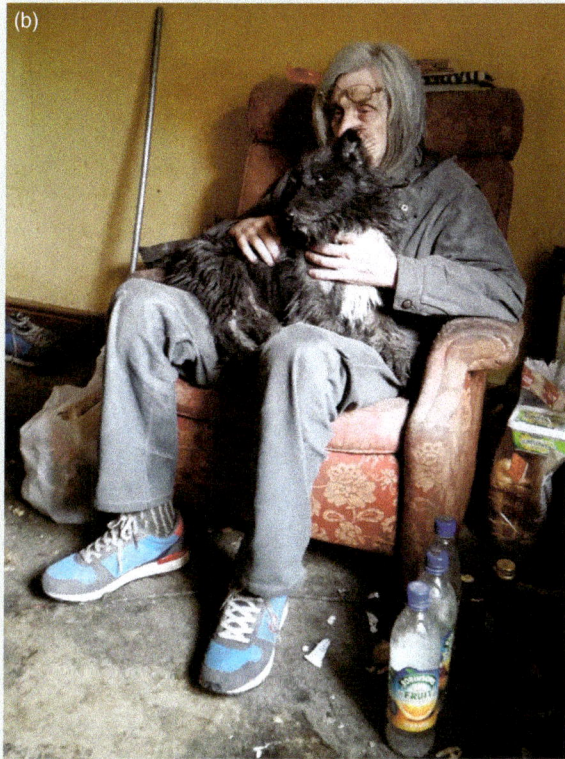

Continued

> **Case Study 7.** Continued.
>
> OSF assessed her needs, and then stayed in regular social contact to monitor her wellbeing and that of Poppy. As her illness progressed, OSF arranged help with dog walking and gave her peace of mind by documenting her wishes for the dog following her death. OSF was able to identify her needs and alert her family and doctor thanks to our regular contact. At the end of her life, she was admitted to a hospice and her family took the dog to visit her while we continued to care for Poppy. The increased social contact experienced by Poppy during her owner's illness enabled her to be rehomed subsequently within the family.
>
> A social worker referred a 68-year-old man who was struggling and living in unsanitary conditions with his beloved sole family member, his dog Billy (image b). OSF initiated ongoing veterinary care for Billy, secured the garden by mending the fencing, and arranged for volunteers to pop in for regular dog walks and a chat. One volunteer was recruited via a weight-reduction club and lost 6 stone while walking Billy. Working alongside health and social carers, the quality of life of Billy's owner improved tenfold and both his welfare and that of Billy were attended to on a daily basis. OSF's intervention meant he could continue to keep his dog at home and, when he was hospitalized as an emergency, Billy was fostered and his owner reassured until they were reunited 8 weeks later.
>
> To date, increasing studies continue to add evidence to the fact that companion animals can help reduce loneliness levels among single people, the elderly and children (Franklin and Tranter, 2011).

Most of the studies published to date, however, tend to focus on the human-positive aspects and health improvements. More work could be done on a holistic approach, considering the animal, human and societal levels. These extend to housing, including social housing, rented accommodation and homes for the elderly.

The animal and human welfare connections can differ greatly at this level. While homelessness has negative impacts both upon those who are homeless and the society that renders them so, dogs owned by homeless people are generally healthy and with few behaviour problems (Williams and Hogg, 2016; Scanlon and Stavisky, 2018).

Through the animal–human bond pets can also help to improve the welfare of homeless people by providing companionship, stability and security, as well as a sense of responsibility. The HAB stages may vary across people; for example it has been reported that the bond between a homeless person and their dog surpasses a typical owner–pet bond and has many similarities with the bond that exists between service or therapy animals and their human counterparts (Scanlon and Stavisky, 2018)

This interconnection is already recognized in a number of countries. As a result multidisciplinary projects to provide food and care for homeless people and their animals at shelters are now in place and established. Studies looking at accommodation availability for homeless people with dogs are ongoing.

Case Study 8 – Vets in the Community (ViC) (by Jenny Stavisky, ViC, England)

The Vets in the Community (ViC) project is based in Nottingham, UK. It was set up in 2012 with the aim of facilitating access to veterinary care for homeless pet owners. Although in the UK there is a strong tradition of charitable veterinary care, accessing free care generally requires an individual to prove they are in receipt of government benefits. For those living outside the social support structure this is a barrier to access. The charitable care available often also focuses on treatment of illness and emergencies, meaning that preventive care (e.g. vaccines and parasite treatments) remains out of reach for many homeless pet owners.

The ViC clinic is run fortnightly and is open to homeless and vulnerably housed individuals who are referred from a network of local services including hostels, drop-in centres, substance abuse treatment facilities and agencies supporting families fleeing domestic abuse. The service is led by students from the University of Nottingham School of Veterinary Medicine and Science (SVMS), under supervision of qualified and experienced veterinary surgeons from SVMS. They provide basic care including health checks, advice, vaccination, parasite control, microchipping and treatment for basic ailments. Where more intensive treatment is needed, referral to other veterinary services is facilitated where possible. Vouchers to cover neutering costs are donated by the Cats Protection and Dogs Trust, and distributed at the clinic sessions.

This project benefits not only the clients but also the students, who gain practical experience in clinical and communication skills. A student committee manages other aspects of ViC. This includes: (i) fundraising, to cover service costs, outreach, pet food and veterinary drug donations; (ii) raising awareness; and (iii) volunteering at each session, to ensure clients are offered a hot drink and homemade cake to make sure they feel welcome and find a warm and inclusive environment.

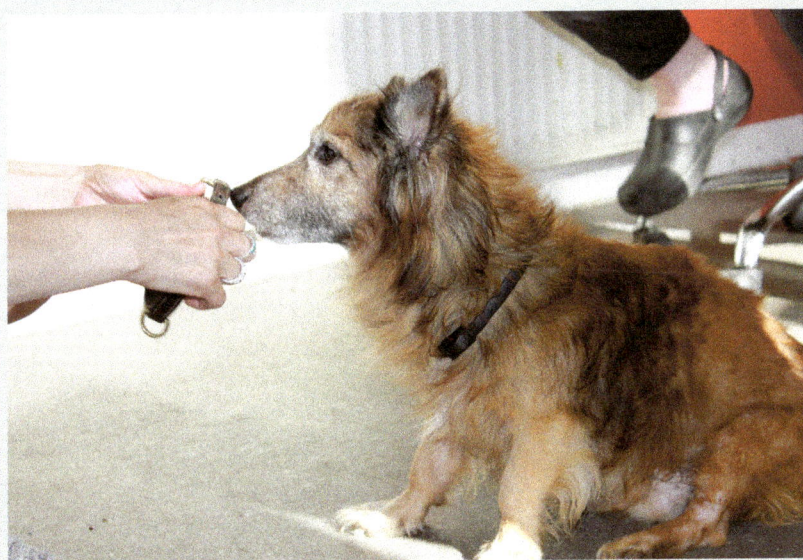

Continued

Case Study 8. Continued.

Clinic sessions are held in the office of *The Big Issue*, a street newspaper from an independent UK-based charity that helps homeless people earn an income; this organization has supported ViC in numerous practical ways over the past 5 years.

Since its inception, the ViC clinic has provided over 1000 consultations and more than 200 students have volunteered their time and services. The benefits to both clients and students have been vast, as shown regularly in the feedback collected. Animal welfare is the main veterinary priority, but the project also considers the strong human–animal relationships between clients and their pets. A parallel research project takes place to characterize this unique HAB. ViC has served as an example to build up similar services across the UK over recent years, and has hosted vets and students from across the UK to share its experiences with them. Homelessness is, unfortunately, prevalent in modern society and pet ownership among homeless people is common, so services like this are necessary to fill a One Welfare gap not yet covered by current organizational structures.

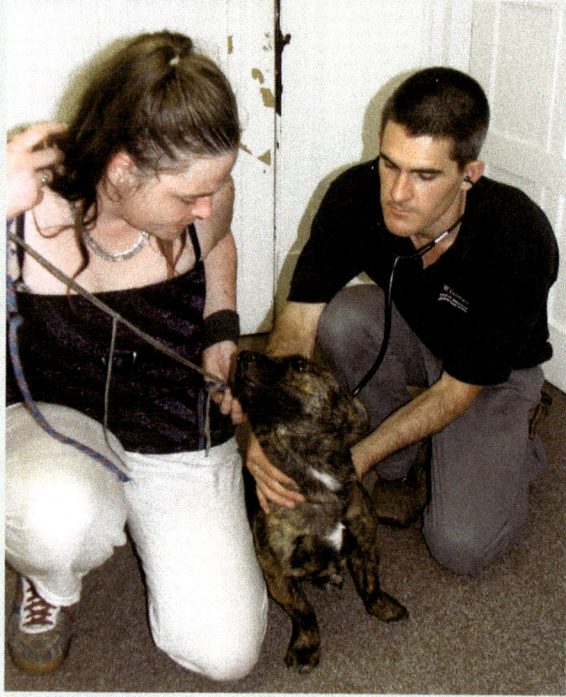

2.2 Working Animals and Livestock Supporting Livelihoods

The benefits of caring well for animals extend to impoverished areas where animal welfare improvements can be an integral part of projects improving human welfare and poverty.

Working animals and livestock play a significant role in rural livelihoods and the economies of developing countries (Herrero *et al.*, 2013). They help with provision of income and employment, and support daily life (traction, transport, etc.). They are especially valuable to pastoralist groups and women, owing to their income generation and contribution to household chores, including transporting feedstuffs and water for other livestock species (Upjohn and Valette, 2014). This is key in regions where public transport or fuel are lacking or very expensive, or where access to either is limited.

The use of working equines such as donkeys or draught horses in poor areas is a good example of interrelations between animals and humans. Better care of the health and welfare of these animals has a direct impact on human health and livelihoods.

Good animal husbandry can directly improve both the welfare of animals and of those who benefit from them, helping provide community support.

The role of the environment also needs to be taken into account. A healthy environment, well managed, can provide a sustainable resource, and this is key to animal welfare, the local community, health, wellbeing and community income.

Case Study 9 – One Welfare in donkey-owning communities in Kenya (by Melissa Liszewski, Brooke) (Case study copyright: Brooke)

Brooke is an international animal welfare organization working to improve the lives of working equids in Africa, Asia, Latin America and the Middle East, as well as of the people who depend on them for their livelihoods. Brooke East Africa's partner, Kenya Network for Dissemination of Agricultural Technologies (KENDAT),

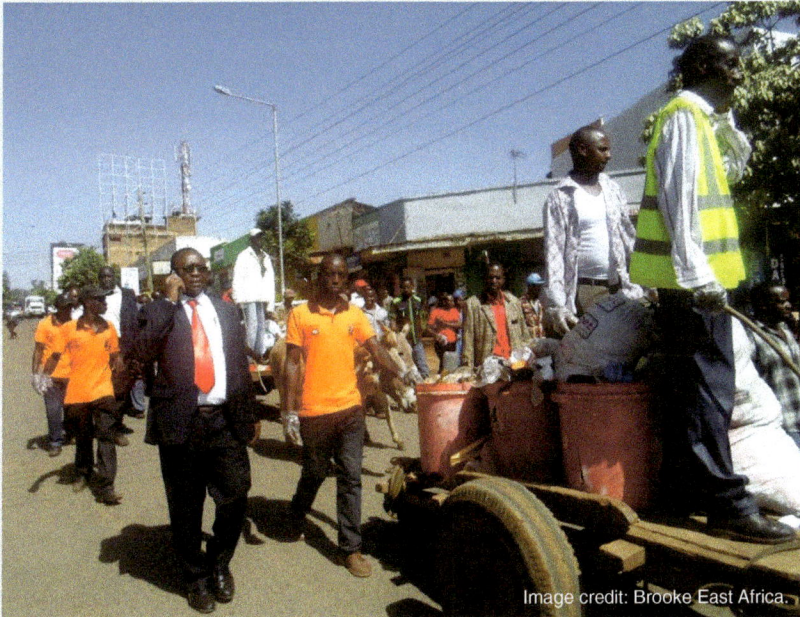

Image credit: Brooke East Africa.

Continued

Case Study 9. Continued.

started working with communities to improve donkey welfare in Meru, Kenya, in 2012. A visit to an association of donkey owners in the area in September 2015 demonstrated the concept of One Welfare in action.

Three years of targeted projects with donkey-owning communities resulted in reductions in wounds, improved local animal healthcare services, and the development and implementation of animal protection by-laws at community group level. These changes protect the animals that countless families across the county depended upon. Leaders of the local donkey welfare groups also described a number of significant human benefits also realized as a result of these projects:

- Increased access to safety nets and support systems: services, advice and opportunities were created to strengthen donkey owners' businesses and to free up capital to be spent on other aspects of their lives. Owners gained access to animal healthcare providers trained in equine medicine, preventative husbandry advice from peer group members, brightly coloured reflective vests to be worn while working on busy roads and loans for emergencies requiring a quick input of cash to preserve or strengthen their donkey business.
  'It is only through the donkey that I finance my family'
  'When we come together in a group we manage to save money'
  'The living standard has been improved'
  'Now we are using the donkey to get the child to university level'
- Increased social status: coming together as a group of professionals to work through shared challenges (animal welfare-related or otherwise) increased the social capital of donkey owners. To improve their image, uniforms were purchased through group savings and bylaws were put in place to protect the animals and people by reducing cart driving while under the influence or alcohol or drugs. The group initiated an annual town clean-up to ensure streets, grazing areas and market places are a safe environment for all, and to remind people how much donkeys and their owners do for the community. Almost 60% of the traders in the market depend on donkeys to transport their produce. Recognition of their contribution by the county government, as well as by the local provincial administration, also boosted the donkey owners' morale and confidence.
  'Before we met these people [KENDAT] even the government saw us as bad people'
  'Even the community knew us as criminals'
  'The rest of the community depends on the donkey'
  'The community now realizes that donkeys are important'
- Fewer conflicts and a platform for local voices to be heard and respected: donkey owners felt empowered for the first time to make their voices heard within their community and beyond; they reported that the number of conflicts and complaints related to donkeys had reduced, and that linking with the government through their groups strengthened their voice even further.

Continued

Case Study 9. Continued.

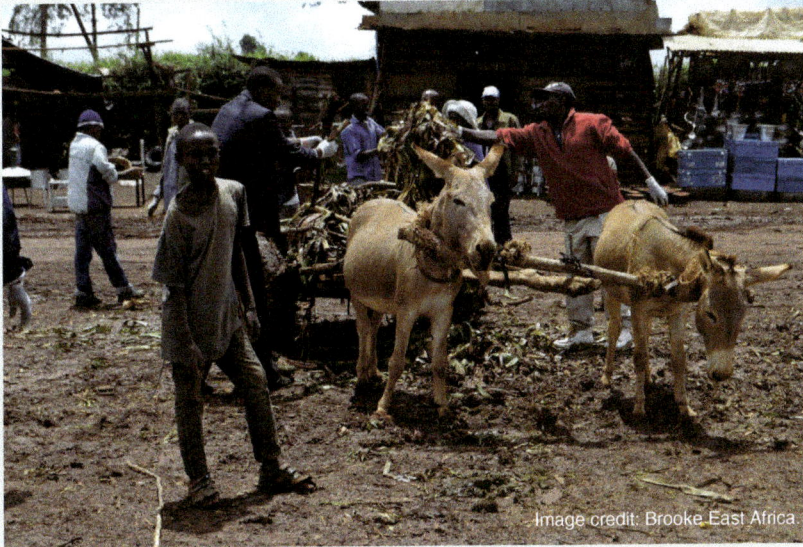

Image credit: Brooke East Africa

KENDAT are working with the Meru donkey owner's groups to build on the progress made so far, as illustrated in the image above, with a key focus over the next few years on developing a better cart and harness design.

> *'[We are] planning to reach nationally and internationally to teach people the importance of this animal'*
> *'We want donkey savings and credit organizations/associations to be all over Kenya'*
> *'[Before] we hated the donkeys and we hated the owner. The donkey owners are now people who are organized. They are people who have a future'.*

These donkey welfare group leaders from Meru, Kenya, demonstrate how a One Welfare approach can simultaneously help to tackle pressing challenges for humans, animals and the environment, delivering impacts that go far beyond what is possible from a silo approach.

(Case study copyright © Brooke)

Management of this subgroup of animals requires engagement with owners at educational and preventative levels, and also with the community to ensure there is an understanding of the essential value they provide (FAO/Brooke, 2011). To support this work it is necessary to build up liaison networks with government agencies, animal welfare organizations, international development departments and environmental organizations, all of which are often not engaged in the process.

It is also important to continue work to develop globally recognized human welfare and poverty indicators; however, the connection with animal welfare indicators is not there yet. To date the use of three groups of indicators: economic, social and enabling environments (Henninger, 1998) has been proposed:

- Economic indicators include measures of current consumption expenditure, income and wealth.
- Social indicators include access to adequate nutrition, energy, education and health, and sanitation services.
- Enabling environments considers important issues such as vulnerability and access to resources and markets.

The Marmot Indicators are another example of wider determinants, also known as social determinants, that include a diverse range of social, economic and environmental factors which impact on people's health (Marmot Indicators, 2017). Correlations with indicators related to animal welfare or human wellbeing are not currently being considered, but could add valuable information and help to improve interventions.

Much of this relates closely to working animals and their roles in supporting humans. Nutritional indicators have also been developed, such as caloric intake or chronic undernutrition (World Food Summit, undated). Undertaking systematic comparisons of such indicators in communities with animals that are well cared for and free of disease could help provide underpinning evidence to a One Welfare, One Health approach.

The role of educational centres and schools can also help to underpin this area by teaching the principles of animal welfare at early educational stages.

2.3   Natural Disasters and War

Natural disasters affect both human and animal welfare through accommodation displacement and reduction in food, water or other environmental resources. Environmental disasters in developing countries, including irregular occupation in urban areas, as well as displacement of local communities in non-urban areas as part of development projects, can also affect both human and animals living in those areas. Equally when there is war both animals and humans can suffer.

Including animals within natural disasters and war interventions is key from a number of different aspects:

- Some humans may be emotionally attached to animals. This could lead to people endangering themselves to protect their animals, or failing to follow public health security procedures, which may lead to a human and animal welfare problem.
- Those dependent on livestock or working animals may be deprived of their source of living and endanger themselves to protect their 'assets', or fall into poverty as a result of damage or death to their animals.
- Welfare impacts on local species can have a deeper effect on the ecosystem and lead to longer-term problems that can be more difficult to resolve.

Case Study 10 – A country at war – conflict often breeds disasters, especially for animals (by Gerardo Huertas, World Animal Protection). (Image credit: © World Animal Protection/Tomas Stargardter.)

Long sections of the border between a country suffering civil war and its neighbours had been planted with landmines during the Civil War. The country is not named here due to the sensitive nature of the topic.

Landmines are war devices that remain active for years, a risk to all living creatures regardless of their species. They are hidden in the ground; vegetation grows and covers any sign of them; and, sometimes, torrential rain moves them to different areas, mainly down slopes. These devices continue to kill innocent victims for years after the conflicts have been resolved.

Many rural families fleeing the war headed towards a neighbouring country and, in trying to do so, took their animals (horses and cattle) with them, as the only assets that could run with them.

Once these families reached the dreaded minefields, they were faced with the dilemma of crossing with their animals, thus increasing the risk of setting one landmine off exponentially, or leaving them behind, and venturing through the 'death fields' by trying to tread in the steps of those who had made it to the other side successfully. 'Every time I have been near or at a minefield the feeling is the same: a giant hole in the stomach, the fear of not knowing what to do, how to step, how to spot them' (anonymous refugee).

Most times, these would-be refugees left their animals tied to trees at the edge of the minefields. After a few days, the desperate animals would start eating the bark of the trees they were tied to, and eventually starve to death.

Local peasants also tried to scare their own pet dogs away but, if they refused to leave, tried to carry them in their arms through the minefields, to prevent them from joyfully following behind and endangering everyone.

The history of these desperate folk and their dying animals was picked up by the local media and, as the government of their country of destination had no jurisdiction over the territory of the country at war, an animal welfare organization took action and arranged a rescue expedition.

Rescuers were able to travel through safe routes to free the surviving horses and cattle, and to carry them safely to the neighbouring country.

This case study highlights how war can affect the innocent, both human and animals. 'I witnessed even worse patterns in other post-war situations, where dairy farms or livestock pastures were being planted with landmines, or homes with pets inside were booby-trapped to target civilians' (anonymous refugee).

Farm animals are essential assets for the livelihoods of civilians who own them and should be off-limits, not only to support livelihoods but also because they are sentient beings. 'Warfare is indeed a nasty type of disaster organized by men that often aims at farm and companion animals as civilian targets' (anonymous refugee).

Increasing the understanding, relief and protection of livestock as essential assets for the livelihoods and wellbeing of those who own them is key, but it is also important to recognize that animals and the environment are undeserving victims of human conflict.

Continued

Case Study 10. Continued.

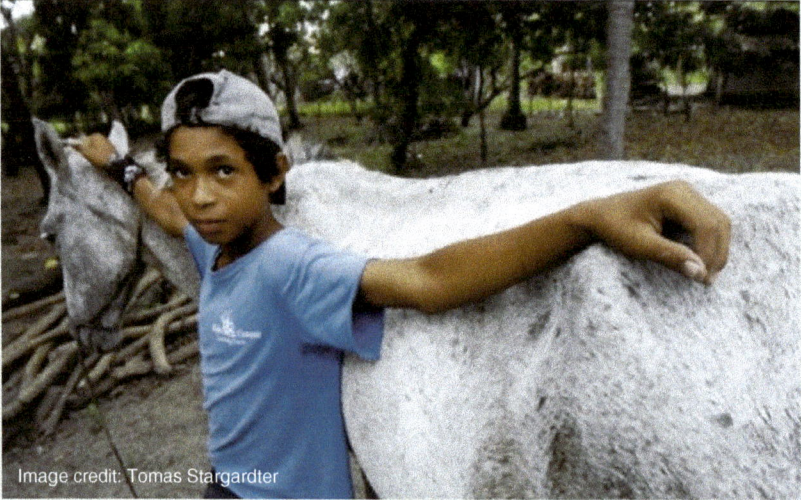

Image credit: Tomas Stargardter

2.4   Animal Welfare and Crime

Awareness of links between the live animal trade, pet ownership and management of social problems extends to criminal behaviour. While most of
the information available in this area is anecdotal, there is growth in the
number of practical cases showing links between animal welfare incidents
and such things as organized animal fights (Levinthal, 2010); use of animals,
such as donkeys, to transport illegal goods like guns or cannabis (ISS, 2010);
or illegal dog breeding and puppy farming.

  This area can overlap with several others mentioned in this book, such as
the links between animal–human abuse and illegal wildlife trade. Although
we are not providing detail in this book, it is important to acknowledge
these connections and to build up an evidence base and case study library
to help develop collaborative frameworks, and to improve effectiveness in
joint work within this complex area.

Case Study 11 – The commercial illegal puppy trade in the UK (by the Royal
Society for the Prevention of Cruelty to Animals, RSPCA)

Between 2012 and 2017 the RSPCA saw a 132% increase in complaints about
the puppy trade to its UK call centre. The increase was mainly the result of
changes to puppy import controls in 2012 and the increased use of the internet
to search for a puppy. Puppy purchasing behaviour is generally an emotional

Continued

Case Study 11. Continued.

response, with 40% of purchasers doing less than a week's research in one poll.[1] The explosion in the use of websites to sell dogs (Gumtree recording a 785% increase in the number of dogs being listed on their site in Great Britain in the past decade) has facilitated large-scale illegal puppy dealing. Of calls the RSPCA receives on animal welfare issues related to the puppy trade, 87% relate to the puppy being bought online.

The illegal puppy trade is an issue that crosses over from animal welfare into other areas such as consumer protection and fraud. This is because the illegal import and sale of puppies is big business. Dealers prosecuted by the RSPCA have been earning around £35,000 a week, or annually near £2 million. Dealers will cross from other illegal activities – such as drugs – to puppies, knowing the financial rewards are similar while the penalties are much reduced.

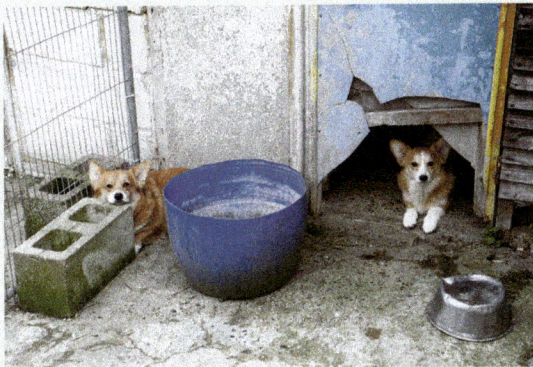

Consumer protection agencies are now starting to look at the fraudulent use of documentation such as vaccination and breeding certificates. Generally, puppy traders and dealers deal in cash only, with no paper trail. This increases the potential for large-scale fraud and results in the loss of large amounts of income to HM Revenue & Customs (HMRC), estimated to extend to tens of millions of pounds annually.

The RSPCA works closely with HMRC to recover undeclared income, and now more

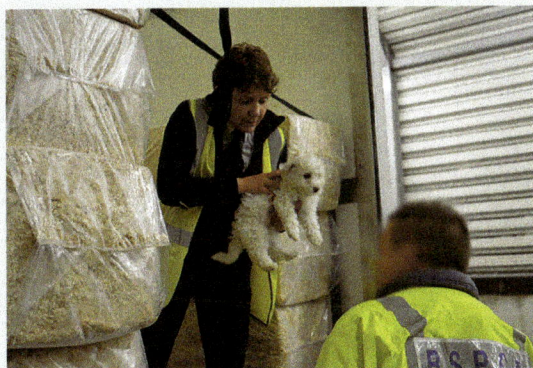

frequently undertakes prosecutions on large-scale puppy dealers under the Proceeds of Crime Act, 2002, and the Fraud Act, 2006, rather than the Animal Welfare Act, 2006. Not only are sentences more severe under the first two Acts, but they also capture the puppy trade as an issue of major crime and loss of income rather than purely an animal welfare problem.

While much is shared about animal welfare issues in the illegal puppy trade, which inevitably leads to the loss of a family pet within days of collection, there

Continued

> **Case Study 11.** Continued.
>
> is now increasing recognition of the linkages between this trade and consumer
> protection, large-scale criminal behaviour and loss of income to the exchequer.
> As a result, these crimes are now taken more seriously by enforcement agencies
> and courts. This inevitably leads to more enforcement effort, a crackdown on
> crime, support for better and clearer legislation and ultimately to an improvement
> in the welfare of the animals being traded.
>
> ¹ TNS 2010. Omnibus Survey for the RSPCA.

2.5 Dealing with the Social Implications of Improved Animal Welfare in Practice

There are now many examples of how multidisciplinary approaches have helped to deliver effective interventions addressing the connections between socio-economic aspects, animal welfare and the environment. While this section does not intend to provide a fully comprehensive summary of globally available tools, we hope that the basic tools and case studies presented will help readers to further investigate, develop, enable or improve collaborative networks and programmes in places where these are not yet in place.

To support work in this area it is key to engage with owners at the educational and preventative level, and also with the community to ensure there is an understanding of the essential value these animals provide. While owners can have an impact on some factors affecting animal welfare, such as the way animals are treated and fed, many other factors such as the people dealing with the animal and the systems in which they both live and work are outside the direct owner's control (van Dijk *et al.*, 2011). Developing One Welfare liaison networks to tackle issues covered in this section should include a number of stakeholders, such as:

- international development departments and environmental organizations;
- educational centres and schools;
- veterinary and animal welfare professionals and other animal service providers;
- animal welfare and protection groups;
- local authority and government representatives;
- social services and other human support services.

Interventions underpinning this section should aim to provide, as a minimum, a local network of key organizations related to the topic. In addition, gathering and facilitating information exchange and education on a number of areas should take place, including:

- data on the local area, and social groups and animals in need of intervention;
- responsible animal ownership;
- animal welfare;
- service providers (vets, welfare professionals, shelters, human services departments etc.).

References

ATSDR (2004) ToxGuide™ for Ammonia NH$_3$. Available at: https://www.atsdr.cdc. gov/toxguides/toxguide-126.pdf (accessed 23 April 2018).

DSM-5 (2013) *Diagnostic and Statistical Manual of Mental Disorders (DSM05)*, 5th edn. American Psychiatric Association, Arlington, VA, USA.

FAO/Brooke (2011) Electronic consultation on the role, impact and welfare of working (traction and transport) animals. http://www.fao.org/fileadmin/user_ upload/animalwelfare/FAO-The%20Brooke%20working%20animals%20e-consultation%20report.pdf (accessed 19 August 2017).

Franklin, A. and Tranter, B. (2011) Housing, loneliness and health. Essay. Australian Housing and Urban Research Institute Southern Research Centre. https://www. ahuri.edu.au/__data/assets/pdf_file/0016/2095/AHURI_Final_Report_No164_ Housing,_loneliness_and_health.pdf (accessed 13 August 2017).

Henninger, N. (1998) *Mapping and Geographic Analysis of Poverty and Human Welfare – Review and Assessment*. Report prepared for the UNEP/CGIAR initia-tive on GIS. World Resources Institute, Washington, DC.

Herrero, M., Grace, D., Njuki, J., Johnson, N., Enahoro, S., Silvestri, S. and Rufino, M.C. (2013) The roles of livestock in developing countries. *Animal* 7(1), 3–18.

ICD (2016) Clutter–Hoarding Scale™. Available at: https://challengingdisorganization. org/resources/clutter-8211-hoarding-scale (accessed 23 April 2018).

ISS (2010) Organised crime in Southern Africa First annual review. Institute for Security Studies, Pretoria, South Africa. https://issafrica.s3.amazonaws.com/site/ uploads/OrgCrimeReviewDec2010.pdf (accessed 22 October 2017).

Johnson, R.A. (2009) Psychosocial and therapeutic aspects of human–animal inter-action. In: Rabinowitz, P.M. and Conti, L.A. (eds) *Human–Animal Medicine. Clinical Approaches to Zoonoses, Toxicants and Other Shared Health Risks*. Saunders, Maryland Heights, MD, USA, pp. 24–36.

Levinthal, J. (2010) The community context of animal and human maltreatment: is there a relationship between animal maltreatment and human maltreatment: does neighborhood context matter? PhD thesis, University of Pennsylvania, PA, USA. http://repository.upenn.edu/edissertations/274 (accessed 19 August 2017).

Marmot Indicators (2017) Marmot Indicators, Public Health England. https://fingertips. phe.org.uk/profile-group/marmot (accessed 22 October 2017).

Mataix-Cols, D. (2014) Hoarding disorder. *New England Journal of Medicine* 370(21), 2023–2030.

NHS (2014) Dog bites: hospital admissions in most deprived areas three times as high as least deprived. http://content.digital.nhs.uk/article/4722/Dog-bites-hospital-admissions-in-most-deprived-areas-three-times-as-high-as-least-deprived (accessed 19 August 2017).

NSA (2016) National Sheep Association, Survey Results. http://www.nationalsheep.org.uk/workspace/pdfs/2016-results.pdf (accessed 7 August 2017).

Patronek, G.J., Loar, L. and Nathanson, J.N. (2006) Animal hoarding: structuring interdisciplinary responses to help people, animals and communities at risk. http://vet.tufts.edu/wp-content/uploads/AngellReport.pdf (accessed 6 August 2017).

Pertusa, A., Frost, R.O., Fullana, M.A., Samuels, J., Steketee, G., Tolin, D., Saxena, S., Leckman, J.F. and Mataix-Cols, D. (2010) Refining the diagnostic boundaries of compulsive hoarding: a critical review. *Clinical Psychology Review* 30(4), 371–386.

Scanlon, L. (2016) Homeless people and their pets – an assessment of animal health and welfare, and the importance of the human–animal bond to vulnerable pet owners. Year 3 research dissertation, School of Veterinary and Medicine Science, University of Nottingham (unpublished).

Scanlon, L. and Stavisky, J. (2018) Homeless people and their pets – an ongoing study into the difficulties of homelessness and pet ownership, health and welfare of pets belonging to homeless owners and the unique bond existing between homeless people and their pets. (Article submitted for publication).

Sylvester, S. and Baranyk, C.W. (2011a) Tales of Justice: When Animal Hoarding is Warehousing for Profit, Part 1. National Center for Prosecution of Animal Abuse, Alexandria, Virginia. Available at: http://www.ndaa.org/pdf/TalesJustice-vol1-no2.pdf (accessed 16 February 2018).

Sylvester, S. and Baranyk, C.W. (2011b) Tales of Justice: When Animal Hoarding is Warehousing for Profit, Part 2. National Center for Prosecution of Animal Abuse, Alexandria, Virginia. Available at: http://www.ndaa.org/pdf/TalesJustice-vol1-no3.pdf (accessed 16 February 2018).

Upjohn, M. and Valette, D. (2014) The relationship between working equids and women in developing countries. *Equine Veterinary Journal* 46 (20). doi:10.1111/evj.12323_46.

van Dijk, L., Pritchard, J., Pradhan, S.K. and Wells, K. (2011) Sharing the Load. https://www.thebrooke.org/sites/default/files/Sharing%20the%20load/SLT%20English/Part-1-English.pdf (accessed 19 August 2017).

Williams, D.L. and Hogg, S. (2016) The health and welfare of dogs belonging to homeless people. *Pet Behaviour Science* (1), 23–30. http://www.uco.es/servicios/ucopress/ojs/index.php/pet/article/view/3998/3913 (accessed 6 August 2017).

World Food Summit (undated) World Food Summit 13–17 November 1996, Rome, Italy. Archived web page. http://www.fao.org/wfs/index_en.htm (accessed 10 February 2018).

Section 3

Animal Health and Welfare, Human Wellbeing, Food Security and Sustainability

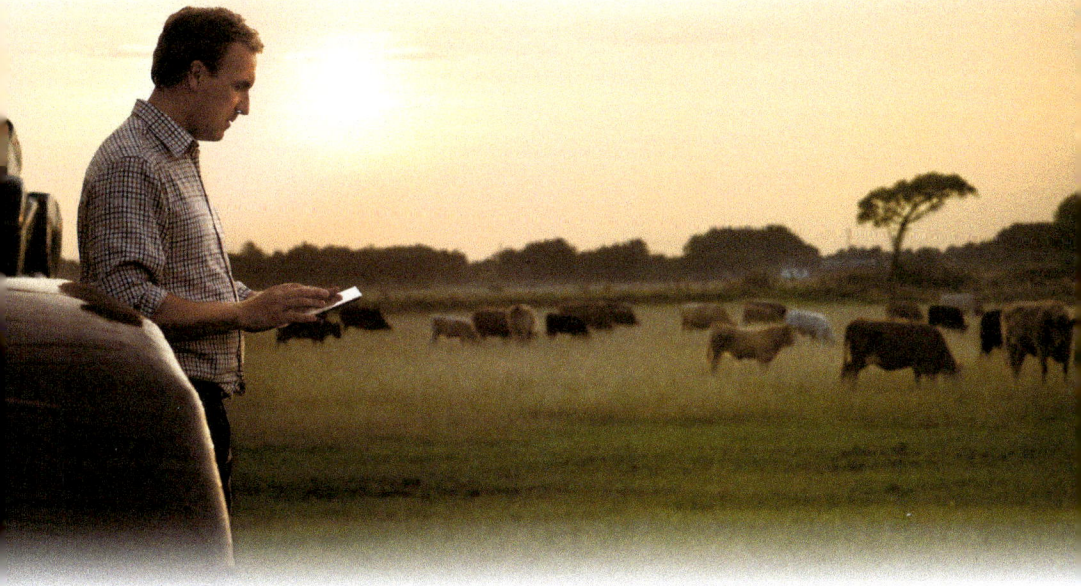

Section 3 of the One Welfare framework includes elements correlating the level of human wellbeing with animal welfare, farming environment and sustainable production practices. It focuses on farming and food-producing livestock, and includes the links between animal welfare and food safety, as well as the beneficial aspects of farm animal welfare improvements to wider areas of societal concern such as climate change, sustainability and global food security.

3.1 Animal Welfare and Food Safety

Improvements in animal welfare have the potential to reduce food safety risks, principally through reduced stress-induced immunosuppression, reduced incidence of infectious disease on farms and reduced shedding of pathogens that can infect humans by farm animals, and through reduced antibiotic use and antibiotic resistance (de Passillé and Rushen, 2005).

Animal welfare has a direct impact on the health of animals and their bacterial content. Food-producing animals may harbour bacteria that can be transmitted to other animals or to humans. Poor animal welfare is a directly contributing factor for increased risk of shedding bacteria, such as *Escherichia coli*, *Salmonella* or *Campylobacter*, in their faeces. This can result in increased risk of cross-contamination, productivity losses due to illness or contamination of meat (Barham *et al.*, 2002; Callaway *et al.*, 2006).

Other studies have shown links between poor animal welfare states, such as stress, as contributory factors to the variable presentation of bacteria such as campylobacteriosis (Cogan *et al.*, 2007).

Considering the type of environment animals are raised in, some studies have reported that free-range and organic systems are examples where improvements to animal welfare – by using an extensive system rather than an intensive indoors one – may expose livestock to increased numbers of bacteria or parasites and hence increase the risk to food safety. They also report that this danger can be reduced or even reversed with adequate risk management, mainly consisting of monitoring and improved management practices (Kijlstra and Bos, 2008; Norwood and Lusk, 2013). Moreover, a range of studies shows that industrial livestock production plays an important part in the emergence, spread and amplification of pathogens (CAST, 2005; Otte *et al.*, 2007). A full review of the different risks and management solutions available is necessary in order to progress.

This means that livestock management practices, including housing, handling and management routines, impact animal welfare and can also affect food safety. For example, a pig study found that increased feed withdrawal times affected the gut microbial ecosystem (the caecal pH increased). Changes in pH could be associated with increased caecal Enterobacteriaceae and *Salmonella* in faeces, which may represent a higher risk of carcass contamination in cases of laceration of viscera (Martín-Peláez *et al.*, 2009). The use of management practices that achieve better animal health and welfare decreases the risk of disease spread and subsequent impacts on food safety. Farms with good animal welfare management have also been found to be, on average, more technically efficient (Czekaj *et al.*, 2013).

> **Case Study 12 – European Food Safety Authority work on animal welfare (by Denise Candiani, European Food Safety Authority)**
>
> The European Food Safety Authority[1] (EFSA) is an agency established in 2002 by the European Union (EU) under the General Food Law – Regulation 178/2002. It provides the EU Commission, Parliament and Member States with independent scientific advice and communication on risks associated with the food chain. Animal welfare is part of EFSA's remit. The safety of the food chain is indirectly affected by the welfare of farmed animals, owing to the close links between animal welfare, animal health and food-borne diseases. EFSA's activities in this field are carried out by a multidisciplinary Panel of experts on animal health and welfare (AHAW). The Panel generally includes academic, government and industry members with expertize on the topic under discussion. Its scientific opinions focus on methods to reduce unnecessary pain, distress and suffering for animals and to increase welfare. The European Commission has mandated the AHAW Panel to provide scientific advice on the welfare of several farm animal categories including pigs, cattle, poultry and fish.
>
> As an example of the work undertaken, in 2017 EFSA and the European Medicines Agency jointly published a scientific opinion on the 'measures to reduce the need to use antimicrobial agents in animal husbandry in the European Union, and the resulting impacts on food safety' (EFSA, 2017). The AHAW Panel contributed to this opinion with a chapter focused on the prevention of disease as a tool to reduce the use of antimicrobials. The need for antimicrobials can be reduced through the application of good farm management and husbandry practices, in particular those aiming at:
>
> - reducing the introduction and spread of microorganisms between farms or within a farm (primary and secondary prevention);
> - increasing the resilience of the animals, namely their ability to cope with pathogens (tertiary prevention).
>
> Tertiary prevention refers to practices that aim to improve animal welfare. It includes appropriate housing, nutrition, stress reduction (by ensuring thermal comfort, reducing stocking density, reducing mixing of unfamiliar animals, ensuring proper weaning, avoiding feed restrictions, ensuring proper animal handling, ensuring proper enrichment, ensuring proper conditions during transport), vaccination and genetic selection. The scientific opinion concludes that 'collectively and individually, these approaches can increase the ability of an animal's immune system to respond appropriately to an infectious challenge' (EFSA, 2017).
>
> [1] EFSA: https://www.efsa.europa.eu/

Another study in broilers in Great Britain showed that *Campylobacter*-positive batches of caeca were associated with higher levels of rejection due to infection and digital dermatitis (Bull *et al.*, 2008). This could mean that interventions to reduce *Campylobacter* levels can also have a positive effect in reducing the prevalence of pododermatitis on target farms, and vice versa.

Illegal meat slaughter also connects to animal welfare and food safety issues as it may lack relevant welfare food inspection safeguards. Collaborations working on the illegal meat trade, welfare aspects and food safety may help to improve intervention efficiency.

Animal feed may also contain elements that can have an impact on both animal welfare and food safety. For example, the presence of toxic metals, pollutants, transmissible spongiform encephalopathies or toxins in animal feed (Fink-Gremmels, 2012) may affect animals consuming such feed as well as impact the safety of the food they produce.

In summary, while not often mentioned, animal welfare and food safety have links that could be explored and disseminated further in a systematic way, to bring a One Welfare approach within this area of public health.

3.2   Improved Animal Welfare and Farmer Wellbeing

This section considers the elements linking farmer wellbeing and animal welfare, including the farming environment and sustainable production practices.

Livestock welfare, farmer wellbeing and their environment are interconnected. This means that improvements in a farmer's wellbeing can lead to improved livestock welfare, and vice versa. Both can be affected by environmental conditions, which include the physical environment, weather conditions,

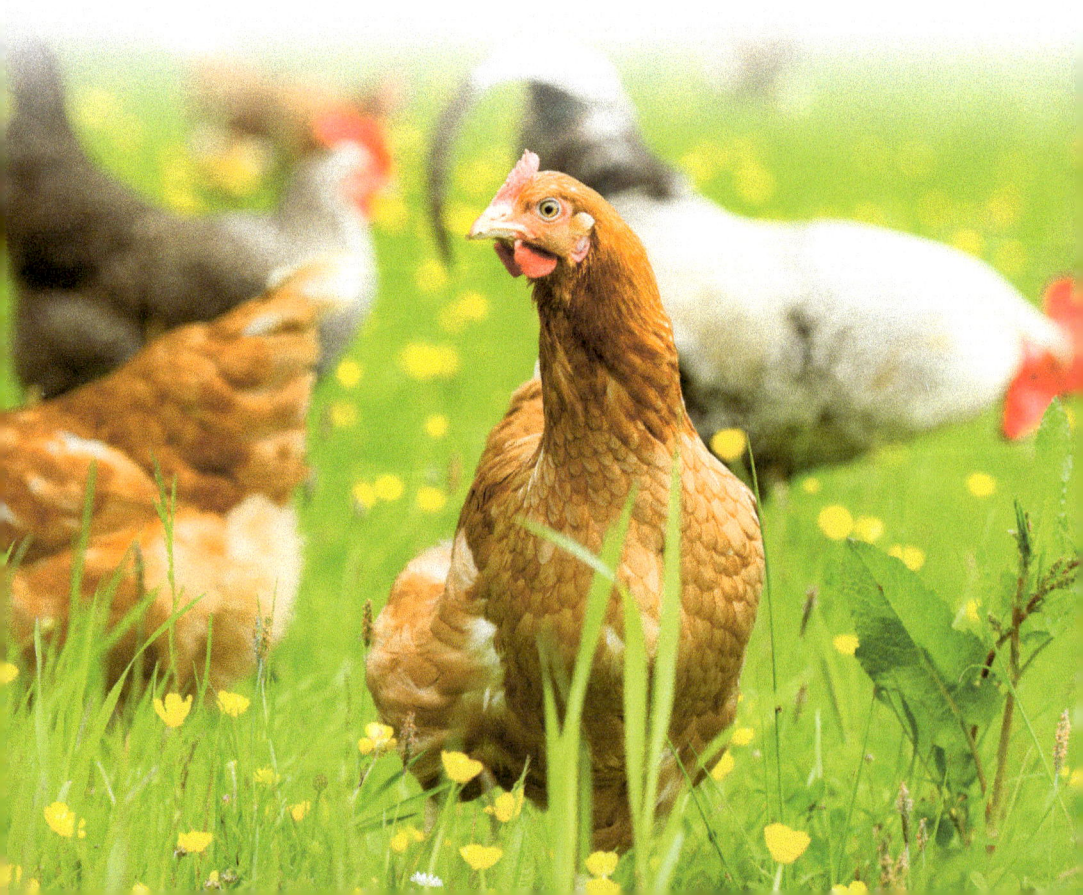

potential for crop and animal diseases or climate-related impacts (Devitt and Hanlon, 2018). Improved animal welfare can result in better farmer job satisfaction and contributions to corporate social responsibility, as well as the ability to command higher prices from consumers (Dawkins, 2017).

Farmers having a good state of health, business, income, social wellbeing and farming knowledge and skills are more likely to provide better husbandry and management practices that result in better animal welfare. Elements such as job satisfaction (Devitt and Hanlon, 2018), peer pressure, trade markets or social concern can have an impact on the wellbeing of farmers. Studies report that social concern has had an effect on the behaviour of farmers that impacts on animal welfare. This may be for economic reasons but may also be due to the attitudes of the farmers and their families, and the public in general (Mazas *et al.*, 2013). The presence of a positive farmer–livestock bond is also important (Devitt and Hanlon, 2018), with variables including how motivated the farmers are and whether they have time available to carry out welfare-oriented tasks (Waiblinger *et al.*, 2006; Kauppinen *et al.*, 2013).

Case Study 13 – Early warning/intervention system (EWS) (by FAWAC, Ireland)

The early warning/intervention system (EWS) is an Irish initiative, introduced in 2004 by the Farm Animal Welfare Advisory Council (FAWAC) involving the central government (Department of Agriculture, Food and the Marine, DAFM); the farming community (Irish Farmers' Association, IFA, and the Irish Creamery Milk Suppliers Association, ICMSA); and the animal protection sector (Irish Society for the Prevention of Cruelty to Animals, ISPCA). The EWS implements the One Welfare approach by providing a framework within which farm animal welfare issues can be identified before they become critical or overwhelming. This has proved to be a very successful animal welfare initiative and the positive approach adopted by its participants has brought greater awareness to the diverse causes of animal welfare problems, allowing intervention at an earlier stage and so preventing chronic welfare scenarios to develop for at-risk animals. EWS is now operating throughout the country.

The role of An Garda Síochána (i.e. the police force of the Republic of Ireland) is also recognized and each Garda division has nominated an identifiable point-of-contact for other participants in the EWS. Other agencies, for example the Health Service Executive (HSE) and private veterinary practitioners, are called upon if they are needed.

The guiding principles of the EWS are that the primary responsibility for the care and welfare of farm animals rests at all times with the farmer. Where actual or potential welfare problems are identified, the earliest possible intervention is desirable, and confidentiality is a fundamental aspect to the success of the EWS.

Two examples of successful scenarios addressed by the EWS follow.

Case 1: Herd Keeper

A single male in his early 40s lived with his 80-year-old mother in an old residence that was in serious disrepair. A phone call to the District Veterinary Office reported that there were dead animals on the farm, and a visit was organized. Dead animals were found and the general situation was one of severe overstocking, no grass, cattle in very poor condition and lack of adequate supplementary feed. The herd

Continued

Case Study 13. Continued.

owner did not have nor was able to provide any more feed at the time, and it was deemed necessary to provide immediate emergency feed for the stock.

The farm had been reduced in size by half when the father died but it still carried the same number of animals. Some of the land was of poor quality. The farmyard and handling facilities were inappropriately located and unsuitable. The herd keeper had a solution for every difficulty identified to him and he had to be persuaded that his solutions were not viable.

An intensive programme was put in place to assist the herd owner to immediately downsize his herd and to provide advice and support to turn around the situation for the long term. The herd owner was fully co-operative and responded very well to the support provided.

Case 2: Herd Keeper

A single female in her early 50s was living alone in very poor living conditions. The holding had been known to DAFM for many years, owing primarily to difficulties in having the required testing programme completed each year. In a deteriorating situation the welfare of the herd was seriously compromised. No animals were sold and they were experiencing health difficulties. Her response was reactionary and obstructive.

Persistence by staff members of DAFM with the aid of the local Garda and the support of the local County Partnership Board, the HSE (health nurse) and the county council helped to bring the situation under control, and she continues to reside in her home. Her herd now comprises three cattle that she looks after with the aid of a relative.

Issues of poor animal health and welfare might be revealing of physical and mental pressures or distress in a farmer (FAWC, 2016). These may drive farmers to a state where they are unable to cope with their farm management for a number of reasons. This may, for example, lead to a negative relationship which can contribute to animal stress, and reduce an animal's ability to produce (Hemsworth and Coleman, 2010). Where poor farmer wellbeing leads to livestock welfare issues, support services and enforcement mechanisms that are able to identify poor states of wellbeing in farming communities are encouraged to work together. This can help to remedy the ongoing human and animal welfare problems, and to prevent future incidents by helping to establish and foster good farming and human wellbeing practices. It is, however, important to recognize that poor animal welfare may not always be connected to poor farmer wellbeing and, in those cases, enforcement action may still be necessary.

The economy of animal welfare in food production is also significant in this context. The power of trade markets and consumers should not be underestimated as they can result in increased or decreased benefits to farming communities. These will then have an effect on their neighbours and the animals they care for. Farmers working in countries with legislation requiring high animal welfare standards may consider this as a prerequisite to their production process. On the other hand, farmers working in countries where neither animal welfare nor legislation has yet reached national consumer awareness may find, for example, that animal welfare improvements can gain them access to export markets and have a positive impact on the number of customers they can reach. This may have an

> **Case Study 14 – Emaciated cattle and severe domestic squalor (by Prairie Mountain Inter-Agency Hoarding Coalition, Canada)**
>
> An elderly farmer with cognitive issues and a lifelong penchant for buying cattle at auction violated an order prohibiting him from acquiring new livestock due to a recent history of neglect. Animal welfare officials intervened and noted that the conditions of the home were squalid and hazardous. Police assisted and transported the individual for mental health assessment. This process resulted in fire and health officials being notified of adverse conditions in the home.
>
> Using relationships established through the animal welfare intervention, permission was obtained from the owner to enter and assess the home. Conditions were such that the home was deemed unfit for occupancy and ordered to be closed under fire and health legislation as there were signs of severe flooding; squalor; imminent fire and health hazards; trip and fall hazards; pest and wildlife infestations; and a multitude of disrepair issues.
>
> Fortunately, the family played a pivotal role in finding safe housing at an assisted-living facility and the individual was able to stabilize and manage his affairs without succumbing in a house fire. This case served as the impetus for establishing an interagency coalition, and a common protocol and resource guide with shared values, goals and objectives. This case study is available online.[1]
>
> ---
> [1] http://www.prairiemountainhealth.ca/images/PublicHealth/PMIHC_Guide1.pdf

impact on farm profits, development and investment in animal welfare and management. Higher welfare labelling schemes have also been mentioned by some as potential drivers for improved farmer income and animal welfare (FAWC, 2011); however, others report that for this to be successful there is a need for positive drivers as well as low consumption barriers (Heerwagen *et al.*, 2013).

Examples of economic factors that are paired with animal welfare include a reduction in labour effort by using welfare-friendly equipment, or improvements in meat quality and productivity margins as a result of good animal welfare and handling (Grandin, 2013). Better animal welfare has direct financial benefits as a result of reduced mortality, improved health, improved longevity for dairy cows, improved product quality, improved resistance to disease, reduced medication, lower risk of zoonoses and animal-borne infections, farmer and producer satisfaction, and higher prices from customers (Dawkins, 2017).

The handling of livestock can be a source of work-related injury and death (FAWC, 2016). Good animal welfare-handling practices can also help reduce these risks by ensuring animals are calmer and more easily handled. These include both the infrastructure for livestock handling and the training, skills and competency of staff handling the animals. Infrastructure not only needs to be adapted to animal behaviour but also to human behaviour, taking into account that working in a non-ergonomic or tiring position with animals that refuse to walk may be quite frustrating (Wiberg, 2012).

While investing in infrastructure for improved handling might be a costly investment, the potential and non-quantified, future benefits of such investment can be as high as a human life. This can be applied to all stages of animal handling, from farm to slaughter.

Stress affects the lactic acid content in muscle and also the keeping ability of meat, having an impact on the quality and eventually profit margins. Conditions that harm animal welfare negatively affect animal health and productivity, and damage specific food quality aspects, thereby jeopardizing profitability and ultimate product quality (Velarde and Dalmau, 2012).

Initiatives that promote increased profitability in farming production systems will and should contribute to welfare improvements. For example, good welfare and health in dairy cows contribute to reduced mortality and improved longevity, which result in reduced costs and increased profits.

While there can at times be some conflicts between animal welfare and efficiency, a One Welfare approach encourages us to explore further and identify areas where better livestock welfare has beneficial effects on a number of areas directly affecting farmers' wellbeing, such as labour satisfaction or overall productivity and profit. While animal welfare and productivity are not always directly correlated, within the same production system animal welfare improvements can often help to improve profit margins and productivity. Livestock with good welfare generally will have better immune systems, which are reflected in decreased levels of disease and lower need for the use of antibiotics (Broom, 2016). This has an indirect effect on the use of antibiotics, and supports the global trend to reduce their use to help prevent antimicrobial resistance, which is becoming a major human and animal health and welfare problem. The disease and health aspects of this section are addressed by ongoing One Health efforts alongside issues where there is a connection between livestock and wildlife disease.

Case Study 15 – The Farming Community Network (by Charles Smith, The Farming Community, Network, England)

The Farming Community Network in England and Wales is a national charity providing pastoral and practical support for farmers and farming families suffering periods of stress and anxiety caused by issues in the farm business or within the family. Such issues may be financial; bureaucratic; or related to physical or mental health, or to animal health and welfare difficulties, relationship breakdowns or disagreements about succession. Frequently, a combination of issues occurs simultaneously to create a seemingly insurmountable barrier to progress (FCN, 2015).

Over the years, strong anecdotal evidence backed up by FCN casework data has confirmed that there is a strong link between animal welfare and farmer wellbeing. This has led many groups to create informal but strong working relationships with other stakeholders such as the Animal and Plant Health Agency (APHA), Trading Standards, the Royal Society for the Prevention of Cruelty to Animals (RSPCA), vets and medical practitioners. These relationships have proved mutually beneficial and led to outcomes that benefitted farmers and animals alike, while helping to avoid costly and often destructive legal interventions.

Continued

> **Case Study 15.** Continued.
>
> This experience has convinced FCN and others that:
>
> - government and its agencies could and should work even more closely with existing farm support networks and commercial and professional organizations, to facilitate early intervention in relation to problems of the poor wellbeing of farm personnel that are having an impact on animal welfare, and vice versa;
> - support networks should be empowered to work more closely together, sharing information and best practice, and making joint decisions on which agency will take responsibility for each case;
> - there should be wider publicity of support networks at different levels, including GP surgeries and veterinary practices and, most importantly, through communications managed by government agencies;
> - government agency staff who interact with farmers should be trained on recognizing both animal and human welfare issues and given guidance on how to respond appropriately.

3.3   Animal Health and Welfare, Environmental Protection, Food Security and Sustainability

This sub-section follows on from sub-section 3.2 to cover the beneficial aspects of livestock welfare improvements to wider areas of societal concern such as climate change, sustainability and food security.

> Food security exists when all people, at all times, have physical, social and economic access to sufficient, safe and nutritious food which meets their dietary needs and food preferences for an active and healthy life. Household food security is the application of this concept to the family level, with individuals within households as the focus of concern.
>
> (FAO, 2003)

Animal welfare is an intrinsic part of sustainable agriculture, and supports food security. However, animal welfare and productivity improvements may actually be counterproductive to sustainability unless they are combined with (i) reduced human consumption of animal products; and (ii) radical changes to animal production that reduce the use for livestock feed components that compete with direct human food (Schader *et al.*, 2015). These include, for example, cereals that can be used more efficiently by humans. In summary, there is a need for both the supply and demand sides – including production and waste – to change if a sustainable food system is to be achieved (Röös *et al.*, 2017).

In ruminant production, good examples of sustainable production systems that can be developed further are those focusing on feed from grassland, such as silvopastoral systems. These include shrubs and trees as well as the more conventional grass pasture. When compared with other ruminant production systems, they can provide efficient feed conversion, increased productivity, higher biodiversity, enhanced connectivity between habitat patches and better animal welfare (Broom *et al.*, 2013). Positive impacts for workers, who like the work and stay in the job longer than people working on conventional farms, have also been reported (Calle *et al.*, 2009). The nutritional quality of the animal feed also impacts on the animal's health and wellbeing, as well as on the meat nutritional content.

There is a link between the economic aspects of farm production, ethical production and food security. There are complex interrelationships between animal welfare issues, economics, climate change, sustainability and food security, and how these may contribute to rethinking consumption habits. This is an area where more can be done to encourage multidisciplinary collaboration and joint work approaches. For example, cross-sectoral studies of human and animal food security would help to develop improved emergency planning for destocking and restocking of livestock in pastoralist production systems (Zinsstag *et al.*, 2015).

The environment, especially the soil and climate, is critical for food security and sustainability. Certain farming production systems can have negative impacts on the environment as a result of, for example, gas emissions, deforestation or soil erosion resulting from intensive feed crop cultivation. More could be done to move towards sustainable farming systems that minimize climate and environmental impacts for the benefit of all.

The availability of natural resources such as land, fossil fuels and water is crucial for livestock farming, in particular to grow crops for animal feed. Few studies, however, recognize or explore these links further, alongside their effects on wild populations, in terms of conservation and the likelihood of infectious hazards which are within the scope of One Health. These aspects could be explored further by using a One Health, One Welfare approach in research and development.

Case Study 16 – Triple wins in milk and beef production (adapted from World Animal Protection, 2014)

The world is facing major challenges developing sustainable livestock production systems that can deliver against growing demands for meat and milk production. These systems must also demonstrate environmental stewardship and ensure that the essential aspects of sustainability, including animal welfare and livelihoods, are properly respected. This case study reveals one such solution: silvopastoral beef and dairy production.

In many Latin American countries, cattle ranching has traditionally relied on extensive systems, with few animals per hectare raised on grass. While it has a range of benefits, this type of cattle ranching provides limited feed quality.

Intensive silvopastoral systems have the potential to deliver much more feed from the land, through the planting of protein- and mineral-rich grasses and shrubs such as *Leucaena* (legume bushes). By growing plants, shrubs and trees, a three-dimensional feed source is created. The quality and quantity of the feed source delivered in situ is greater. The additional plant matter (plus root density) and biodegradable material can increase soil quality and water retention, as well as increasing carbon retention in the soil.

Continued

Case Study 16. Continued.

By using animal breeds well adapted to tropical environments, the intensive silvopastoral system has the potential to achieve high levels of production from local feed sources in pasture-based environments. This maintains good health and welfare, natural behaviour and ease of animal management. A 2014 review of an example project in Colombia aimed to bring together measures of productivity, economics (and the potential for livestock-based livelihoods), environmental stewardship and animal welfare into one integrated assessment. This novel project aimed to test the potential of an alternative system, and its development over time to achieve sustainable livestock production. The assessment was delivered as a partnership project between partners including the Colombian Cattle Ranching Association (FEDEGAN-FNG); the Centre for Research on Sustainable Agricultural Production Systems (CIPAV); the global assessment network agri benchmark of the Thünen Institute of Farm Economics; and World Animal Protection.

The project assessed three different areas:

- Productivity: the analysis of the production system, productivity and economics used the tools, methods and expertize of the global, non-profit agri benchmark Beef and Sheep Network.
- Environment: intensive silvopastoral systems provide enhanced habitat and food resources for birds, mammals and invertebrates owing to the structural and biological complexity with several species of grass, shrubs and trees. Deep-rooted trees contributed to the recovery of nutrients and water from deeper soil layers, increasing tolerance to drought and to biomass production and carbon sequestration both below and above ground.
- Animal welfare: cattle welfare was assessed on each of three farms and the results were compared with those from a farm using standard cattle ranching systems. The assessment took direct measures of feed and water availability, behaviour, heat stress, body condition and evidence of parasites.
- The farms assessed are pioneers in establishing intensive silvopastoral systems, delivered with the technical and scientific support of CIPAV. This has proved crucial for the development and dissemination of the systems.

The results of this case study showed that intensive silvopastoral systems:

- are more productive and profitable than conventional cattle ranching systems. The silvopastoral systems measured had higher milk yields in cows and higher daily weight gains in finishing cattle, allowing a reduction in finishing periods and an increase in cattle numbers. Their success is based on good management, extension and access to capital that builds farmers' long-term capacity to deliver efficient and increasingly productive beef and dairy production;
- deliver productivity that goes hand in hand with good animal health and welfare. The environmental design of the system provides good-quality green forage (not usable as food for humans) to meet animals' nutritional needs. Water is provided freely, and trees and shrubs provide shade, which is important for cow comfort and to prevent heat stress. Animals also have freedom of movement and can exhibit natural behaviours;
- provide a clear investment in sustainable environmental management, with potential climate mitigation benefits.

3.4   One Welfare within Production Systems in Practice

Putting aspects of One Welfare into practice within food production systems requires collaborative networks to be set up.

For example, using sustainability as the basis, a fully comprehensive approach could include eight different areas to assess sustainability in livestock production systems: animal welfare, animal health, breeding programmes, environment, meat safety, market conformity, economy and working conditions (Bonneau *et al.*, 2014).

Collaborative approaches around this section can focus on at least at three different levels:

- **Farmer support networks:** these can focus on farmer wellbeing with links to animal welfare organizations or government inspectorates.
- **Farm welfare enforcement networks:** these are mainly focused on farm welfare inspections, but with links to community support organizations, to ensure that the wellbeing of farmers can be identified, supported and addressed if necessary.
- **Multi-agency groups:** these are linked to animal welfare data surveillance during farm visits, transport and at slaughter. These groups will comprise organizations related to on-farm inspections, livestock transport and slaughter facilities, to ensure animal welfare issues are systematically monitored, reported and linked through the production chain in an efficient and effective manner.

In relation to enforcement networks, these can link closely with animal health service provision for maximum efficiency and a fully comprehensive One Health, One Welfare approach. The list below includes areas suggested as core functions of animal health services (FAO, 2002). Animal and human welfare elements can also be integrated within these functions, and so some of the bullet points have been modified to reflect this:

- ministerial briefing and support;
- planning, coordination and implementation of animal welfare and national disease-control programmes;
- animal welfare and disease surveillance and other early warning measures, epidemiological analysis and disease reporting at national and international levels;
- risk analysis as an input to quarantine, health and welfare surveillance, contingency planning and priority setting;
- quarantine and animal-movement controls;
- veterinary public health and food safety, with regard to the animal welfare aspects in these areas;
- preparedness for high-threat epidemic diseases including humane control measures;

- international and regional liaison and cooperation;
- licensing of vaccines and drugs;
- close liaison with farmers' groups and private-sector animal-health and human support services;
- quality assurance of public and private animal health and welfare services.

Some key areas where support networks can provide resources are shown in the following list (the last five bullet points are adapted from FAO, 2002). They could enable:

- Identification of farmer wellbeing issues (FCN, 2015).
- Provision of contact details for support services.
- Communication and alert networks for professionals visiting farms occasionally (vets, auditors, neighbouring farmers, etc.).
- Identification of poor animal and human welfare issues.
- Analysis of data to assist any of the above by triggering early-warning systems which can enable early-stage support mechanisms to both farmers and animals.
- Use and development of people's abilities and skills to analyse and evaluate their surroundings, including the livestock and their environment.
- People to analyse their situations and see how human, animal and environmental resources are being used efficiently and effectively, thus setting local priority needs.
- People to study their own methods of animal care, production and management.
- An increase in the sense of collective responsibility for implementation, monitoring and evaluation.

References

Barham, A.R., Barham, B.L., Johnson, A.K., Allen, D.M., Blanton Jr, J.R. and Miller, M.F. (2002) Effects of the transportation of beef cattle from the feedyard to the packing plant on prevalence levels of *Escherichia coli* O157 and *Salmonella* spp. *Journal of Food Protection* 65, 280–283.

Bonneau, M., Klauke, T.N., Gonzàlez, J., Rydhmer, L., Ilari-Antoine, E., Dourmad, J.Y., de Greef, K., Houwers, H.W.J., Cinar, M.U., Fàbrega, E., Zimmer, C., Hviid, M., van der Oever, B. and Edwards, S.A. (2014) Evaluation of the sustainability of contrasted pig farming systems: integrated evaluation. *Animal* 8(12), 2058–2068.

Broom, D.M. (2016) Animal Welfare in the European Union. Available at: http://www.europarl.europa.eu/RegData/etudes/STUD/2017/583114/IPOL_STU(2017)583114_EN.pdf (accessed 21 August 2017).

Broom, D.M., Galindo, F.A. and Murgueitio, E. (2013) Sustainable, efficient livestock production with high biodiversity and good welfare for animals. *Proceedings of the Royal Society B* 280(1771), 2013–2025.

Bull, S.A., Thomas, A., Humphrey, T., Ellis-Iversen, J., Cook, A.J., Lovell, R. and Jorgensen, F. (2008) Flock health indicators and *Campylobacter* spp. in commercial housed broilers reared in Great Britain. *Applied and Environmental Microbiology* 74, 5408–5413.

Callaway, T.R., Morrow, J.L., Edrington, T.S., Genovese, K.J., Dowd, S., Carroll, J. *et al.* (2006) Social stress increases fecal shedding of *Salmonella* Typhimurium by early weaned piglets. *Current Issues in Intestinal Microbiology Journal* 7, 65–71.

Calle A., Montagnini F. and Zuluaga A.F. (2009) Farmers' perceptions of silvopastoral system production in Quindio, Colombia. *Bois et Forets des Tropiques* 300, 79–94.

CAST (2005) Council for Agriculture, Science and Technology. Global Risks of Infectious Animal Diseases. Issue Paper 28. pp.15. Available at: http://www.cast-science.org/download.cfm?PublicationID=2900&File=f030f5b5845ecc35e2b0631a124043596147(accessed 31 October 2017).

Cogan, T.A., Thomas, A.O., Rees, L.E., Taylor, A.H., Jepson, M.A., Williams, P.H. *et al.* (2007) Norepinephrine increases the pathogenic potential of *Campylobacter jejuni*. *Gut* 56, 1060–1065.

Czekaj, T.G., Nielsen, A.S., Henningsen, A., Forkman, B. and Lund, M. (2013) The relationship between animal welfare and economic outcome at the farm level. Department of Food and Resource Economics, University of Copenhagen. http://curis.ku.dk/ws/files/56173245/IFRO_Report_222.pdf (accessed 21 August 2017).

Dawkins, M.S. (2017) Animal welfare and efficient farming: is conflict inevitable? *Animal Production Science* 57, 201–208.

Devitt, C. and Hanlon, A. (2018) Farm animals and farmers: neglect issues. In: Day, M.R., McCarthy, G. and Fitzpatrick, J.J. (eds) *Self-Neglect in Older Adults: a Global, Evidence-Based Resource for Nurses and Other Healthcare Providers*. Springer, New York, pp. 69–81.

EFSA (2017) EMA and EFSA joint scientific opinion on measures to reduce the need to use antimicrobial agents in animal husbandry in the European Union, and the resulting impacts on food safety (RONAFA). *EFSA Journal* 15(1), DOI 10.2903/j.efsa.2017.4666. Available at: https://www.efsa.europa.eu/en/efsajournal/pub/4666 (accessed 10 February 2018).

FAO (2002) Improved animal health for poverty reduction and sustainable livelihoods. FAO Animal Production and Health Paper 153. Food and Agriculture Organization of the United Nations, Rome Available at: http://www.fao.org/docrep/005/Y3542E/y3542e00.htm#Contents (accessed 1 October 2017).

FAO (2003) *Trade reforms and food security, conceptualizing the linkages*. FAO, Rome, Italy, pp. 25–34. Available at: http://www.fao.org/3/a-y4671e.pdf (accessed 16 February 2018).

FAWC (2011) Economics and farm animal welfare. Farm Animal Welfare Council, London. Available at: https://www.gov.uk/government/uploads/system/uploads/attachment_data/file/324964/FAWC_report_on_economics_and_farm_animal_welfare.pdf (accessed 10 February 2018).

FAWC (2016) Opinion on the links between the health and wellbeing of farmers and farm animal welfare. Available at: https://www.gov.uk/government/uploads/system/uploads/attachment_data/file/593474/opinion-on-farmer-wellbeing_final_2016.pdf (accessed 21 August 2017).

FCN (2015) Fit for farming. Available at: https://issuu.com/menshealthforum/docs/fit_for_farming_2015_hr (accessed 21 August 2017).

Fink-Gremmels, J. (2012) *Animal Feed Contamination: Effects on Livestock and Food Safety*. Woodhead Publishing Limited, Cambridge, UK.

Grandin, T. (2013) The effect of economics on the welfare of cattle, pigs, sheep, and poultry. Available at: http://www.grandin.com/welfare/economic.effects.welfare.html (accessed 21 August 2017).

Heerwagen, L.R., Christensen, T. and Sandøe, P. (2013) The prospect of market-driven improvements in animal welfare: lessons from the case of grass milk in Denmark. *Animals* 3(2), 499–512. Available at: http://www.mdpi.com/2076-2615/3/2/499/htm (accessed 24 September 2017).

Hemsworth, P.H. and Coleman, G.J. (2010) *Human–Livestock Interactions: The Stockperson and the Productivity and Welfare of Intensively Farmed Animals*, 2nd edn. CAB International, Wallingford, UK.

Kauppinen, T., Valros, A. and Vesala, K.M. (2013) Attitudes of dairy farmers toward cow welfare in relation to housing, management and productivity. *Anthrozoos* 26, 405–420.

Kijlstra, A. and Bos, A.P. (2008) Animal welfare and food safety: danger, risk and the distribution of responsibility. 16th IFOAM Organic World Congress, Modena, Italy, June 16–20 2008. Available at: http://orgprints.org/12253/1/12253.pdf (accessed 21 August 2017).

Martín-Peláez, S., Peralta, B., Creus, E., Dalmau, A., Velarde, A., Pérez, J.F. *et al.* (2009) Different feed withdrawal times before slaughter influence caecal fermentation and faecal *Salmonella* shedding in pigs. *The Veterinary Journal* 182, 469–473.

Mazas, M., Manzanal, R.F., Zarza, F.J. and María, G.A. (2013) Development and validation of a scale to assess students' attitude towards animal welfare. *International Journal of Science Education* 35 (11), 1775–1779.

Norwood, F.B. and Lusk, J.L. (2013) Animal welfare and food safety. Available at: http://www.foodsafetymagazine.com/magazine-archive1/februarymarch-2013/animal-welfare-and-food-safety/#References (accessed 21 August 2017).

Otte, J., Roland-Holst, D., Pfeiffer Soares-Magalhaes, R., Rushton, J., Graham, J., and Silbergeld, E. (2007) Industrial livestock production and global health risks. Food and Agriculture Organization of the United Nations, Pro-Poor Livestock Policy Initiative Research Report. Available at: http://citeseerx.ist.psu.edu/viewdoc/download;jsessionid=6AD5121C8407B600826E692895FEC61B?doi=10.1.1.114.1119&rep=rep1&type=pdf (accessed 3 October 2017).

de Passillé, A.M. and Rushen, J. (2005) Food safety and environmental issues in animal welfare. *Scientific and Technical Review of the Office International des Epizooties (Paris)* 24(2), 757–766. Available at: http://www.oie.int/doc/ged/D2708.PDF (accessed 15 October 2017).

Röös, E., Bajželj, B., Smith, P., Patel, M., Little, D. and Garnet, T. (2017) Greedy or needy? Land use and climate impacts of food in 2050 under different livestock futures. *Global Environmental Change* 47, 1–12. Available at: http://www.sciencedirect.com/science/article/pii/S0959378016306872 (accessed 1 October 2017).

Schader, C., Muller, A., El-Hage Scialabba, N., Hecht, J., Isensee, A., Erb, K.-H., Smith, P., Makkar, H.P.S., Klocke, P., Leiber, F., Schwegler, P., Stolze, M. and Niggli, U. (2015) Impacts of feeding less food-competing feedstuffs to livestock on global food system sustainability. *Journal of the Royal Society Interface* 12 20150891. DOI: 10.1098/rsif.2015.0891. Available at: http://rsif.royalsocietypublishing.org/content/12/113/20150891 (accessed 30 September 2017).

Velarde, A. and Dalmau, A. (2012) Animal welfare assessment at slaughter in Europe: moving from inputs to outputs. *Meat Science* 92, 244–251.

Waiblinger, S., Boivin, X., Pedersen, V., Tosi, M-V., Janczak, A.M., Visser, E.K. and Jones, R.B. (2006) Assessing the human–animal relationship in farmed species: A critical review. *Applied Animal Behaviour Science* 101, 185–242.

Wiberg, S. (2012) Slaughter – not only about animals. An interdisciplinary study of handling of cattle at slaughter. Licenciate thesis, Swedish University of Agricultural Sciences, Skara, Sweden.

World Animal Protection (2014) A case study of triple wins in milk and beef production in Colombia. Available at: https://unfccc.int/files/documentation/submissions_from_non-party_stakeholders/application/pdf/521.pdf (accessed 1 February 2018).

Zinsstag, J., Schelling, E., Waltner-Toews, D., Whittaker, M. and Tanner, M. (eds) (2015) *One Health: The Theory and Practice of Integrated Health Approaches*. CAB International, Wallingford, UK.

Section 4

Assisted Interventions Involving Animals, Humans and the Environment

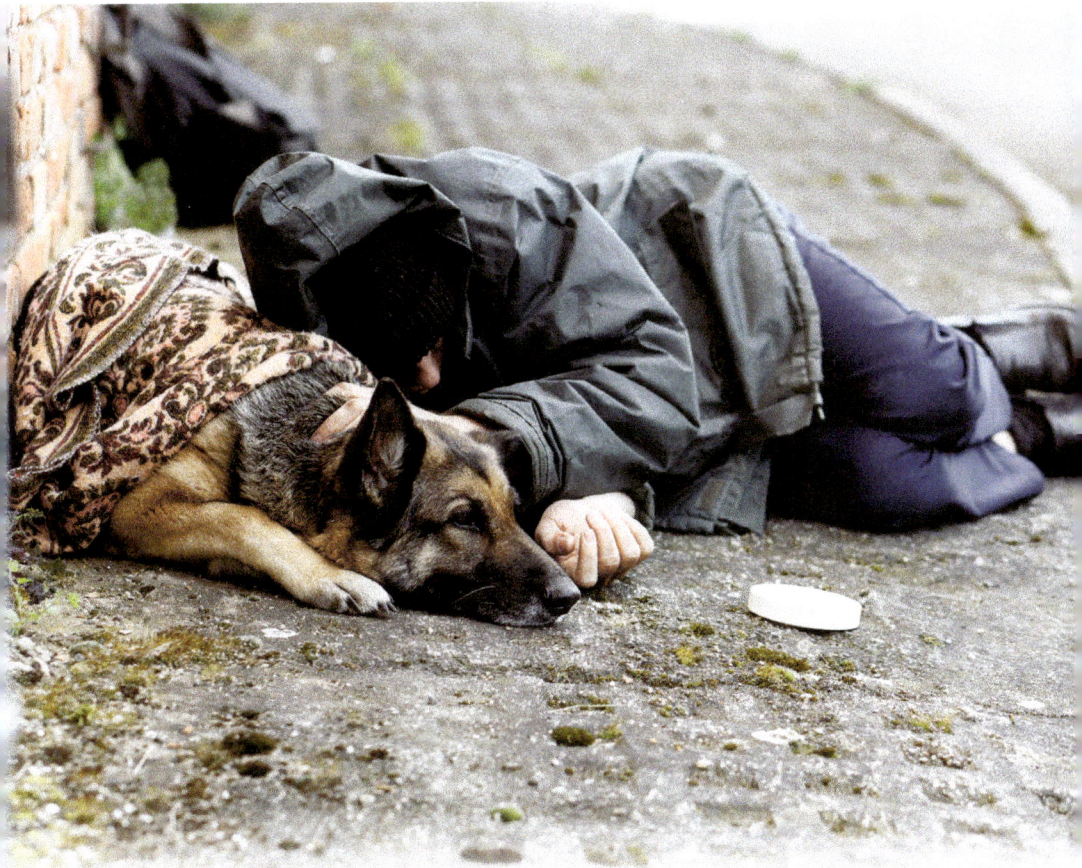

Section 4 of the One Welfare framework describes those activities involving animals, humans and the environment that involve a need for support, rehabilitation and managed animal rehoming programmes. It highlights and encourages forms of such work that take into consideration the benefits for all the parties involved.

At times, animals, humans and the environment are in need of interventions to support their wellbeing. While they are interdependent, each element is independent of the others, and sometimes interventions can help one while harming another. We should strive to prioritize interventions that benefit all. Interventions can aim to address both the chance for life and the chance for a better quality of life for the parties involved. With a growing body of research supporting the benefits of human–animal interactions (HAI) and the human–animal bond (HAB), assisted interventions involving both humans and animals are increasing.

To date, interventions and research have had a strong focus on positive impacts on humans with little investigation of potential positive or negative impacts on animals or the environment. A literature review has reported that some evidence is available on the impact of interventions in agricultural animals (Hosey and Melfi, 2014). It is important for research studies and interventions to take a comprehensive approach, looking at the environmental impacts of HAI, as well as the impacts of HAI and the HAB on animals. Section 4 aims to reinforce the thinking that we should aim for assisted interventions that promote a mutual benefit for humans, animals and the environment.

4.1   Interactions Between Humans, Animals and the Environment

The term 'Green Care' has been proposed as an inclusive term for many 'complex interventions' including care farming, therapeutic horticulture and others that promote physical and mental health and wellbeing through interactions between humans, animals and the environment (Sempik *et al.*, 2010). Although to date interventions seem to focus either on the benefits of interactions between humans and the environment or the impact between humans and animals, few interventions use a combination of all three. Information on whether combined approaches would have greater beneficial impact on humans, animals and the environment is not yet available. There is scope to explore a One Welfare approach to Green Care that combines all these aspects.

> **Case Study 17 – Green Chimneys (by Green Chimneys, USA)**
>
> Green Chimneys, a nonprofit education and human services agency based in New York, USA, helps young people to maximize their potential by providing residential, educational, clinical and recreational services in a safe and supportive environment that nurtures connections with their families, the community, animals and nature, using a One Welfare approach.

Continued

Case Study 17. Continued.

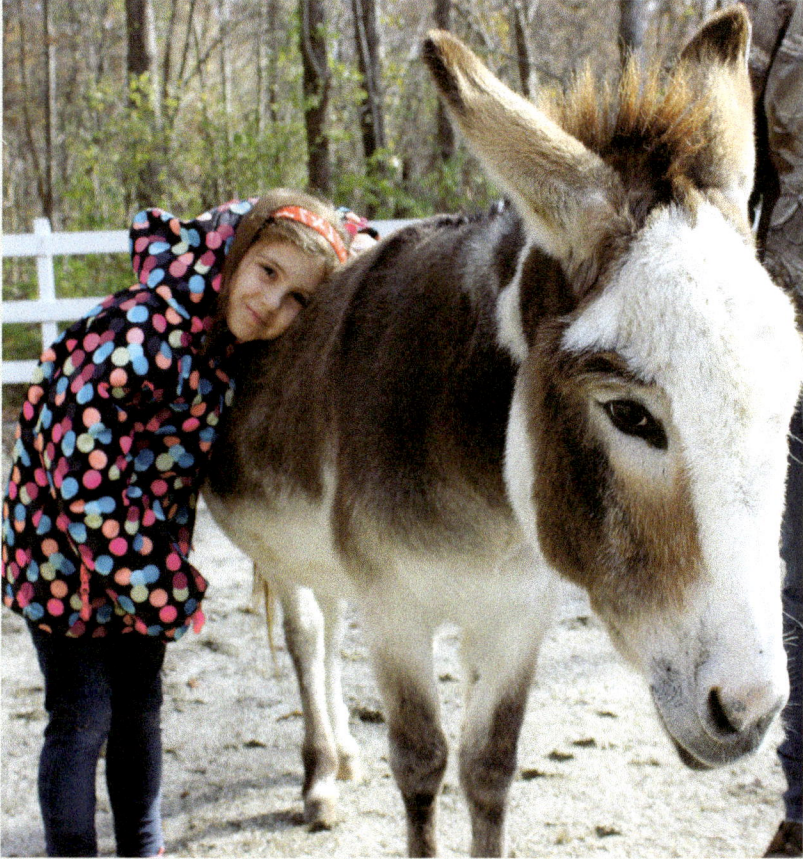

Established in 1947, Green Chimneys offers therapeutic education, environmental and recreation programmes, and clinical treatment including animal-assisted therapy for children with social, emotional and behavioural challenges. The interconnection of human wellbeing, animal welfare and environmental stewardship is ingrained in the organization's founding principles.

The organization's philosophy is based on the belief that, if children are given a chance to explore and discover their inherent strengths in a safe and structured nature-based environment, their self-esteem, compassion, coping and social skills will improve. The concept of an enriched treatment setting that brings people together with animals and plants in a mutually beneficial relationship lies at the heart of Green Chimneys' founding principles.

Its approach focuses on an awareness of how trauma impacts human and animal lives, that a healing setting can benefit both, and that there is a broader parallel between human, animal, environmental and societal wellbeing. Human–animal contact, and contact with all aspects of nature, can have a profound effect on

Continued

Case Study 17. Continued.

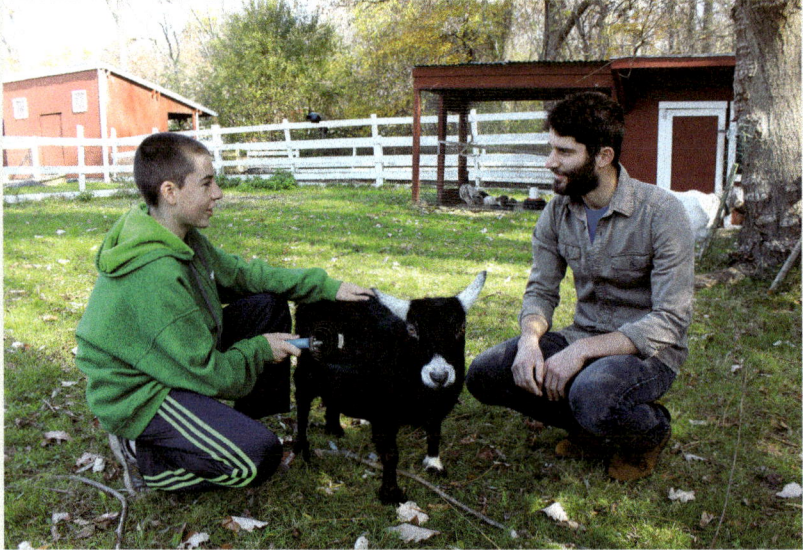

people. These elements are an integral part of the Green Chimneys physical facilities and organizational identity.

Animal welfare is at the core of the Green Chimneys mission and great efforts are made to provide optimal nutrition, housing and veterinary care for the animals involved. The role of the farm animals, horses and other species at Green Chimneys is to live in a mutually beneficial relationship. The animals of the Farm and Wildlife Center are valued partners, and staff members aim to ensure that animals benefit as much from the interactions as the children do. Resident animals are not objects to be used, but individuals to interact with in a respectful manner. Most importantly, the students learn to become the caretakers of these animals and the shared environment.

Children can respond to animals in ways in which they often cannot do with people. The human–animal contact helps bring out a nurturing instinct in children. Learning to care for animals fosters a sense of responsibility and empathy among children who may not have experienced this themselves. Interactions range from playing with a dog, cat or rabbit during a session with a trained adult, to a more comprehensive approach where children experience an immersion with animals or nature, including therapeutic horseback riding, horticulture therapy including greenhouse and garden work, outdoor adventure activities, and a dog interaction and training programme to help prepare rescued dogs for adoption.

Most children come to the Farm and Wildlife Center in their first days with their social worker, class or dorm staff. They soon 'pick out' a favourite animal quite naturally, and the child is given opportunities to work with that animal and form a bond. However, all the animals are shared by everyone and they are all to be taken care of; the child's desire to care for 'their' animal dictates that they learn about that animal from others. The trust and friendship established because of the animal's needs and the child's desire to nurture it are often the basis for therapeutic treatment; the animal acts as a bridge from the child to the staff working to help them become successful.

4.2   Benefits of the Human–Animal Bond (HAB)

Many publications describe the physical, mental and socio-economic bene-fits of appropriate, well-matched and supported human–animal relationships. Some describe in detail the factors connected to improved wellbeing that can lead to support in recovery from major illness, prevention of ill-health, enhanced social interactions, improvements to self-esteem, elevated mood, increased mental resilience or fewer visits to the doctor. Overall this results in wider community and societal benefits, from con-tributions in the form of savings to wider healthcare expenditure, or to improvements to the local social community (Clower and Neaves, 2015; Hall *et al.*, 2017).

Practical case studies show how social isolation and general physical and mental frailty can be supported by companion animal ownership, in a way that offers mutual positive benefits. However, it is important to note that interactions need to be managed and properly resourced to prevent negative effects. These may include deferral of important surgery or hospitalization; deferring spending money on the owners' health for the sake of a pet or fear that an animal may be hurt or die if unattended; or failure to evacuate in an emergency situation through fear for their animal's safety (Hunt *et al.*, 2012). Other negative effects that can impact on human wellbeing may include being woken in the night (Christiansen *et al.*, 2013).

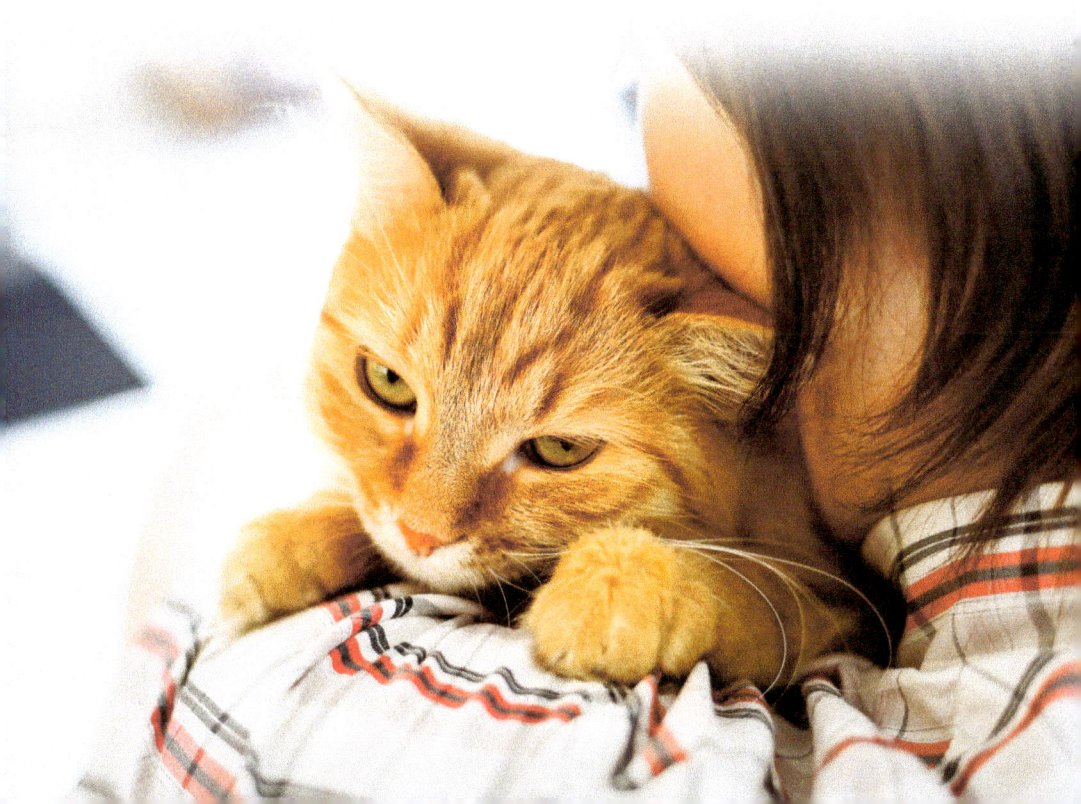

From a medical point of view is important to assess the patient's physical and cognitive functions and to ensure that they have sufficient support systems (e.g. home helpers or family) to enable the proper care of the animal (Johnson, 2009). Some non-governmental organizations (NGOs) working in this area are coming across issues related to 'invisible frailty'. Targeted interventions can help to make these issues visible to available community support but, for this to happen, such interventions need to be enabled.

There are also societal aspects of pet companionship and its positive effects on human wellbeing. Cohabiting with pets may, for example, encourage humans to care more about animals and nature; or it may encourage them to interact with other people in their community, promoting – where animals are kept responsibly – positive social interactions. Overall, they contribute towards the social capital of communities, and many times also help people to get in touch with each other and so help to foster a community spirit (Mills, 2012). While the positive effects of companion animals on human health and welfare are well documented, it is important to note that there may be negative effects in some cases, although to date these have not been widely reported.

Assisted intervention programmes may include a wide range of animals, although most appear to be undertaken with dogs, horses and farm animals. Much of the focus of such interventions is on the human benefits (e.g. Friedmann and Son, 2009), but more needs to be done to understand whether the animals also benefit from these interactions, so that mutually beneficial One Welfare interventions can be made. Examples of existing intervention programmes that are already taking place across the world include:

- **Animal-assisted intervention (AAI)**, an overarching term that encompasses all different intervention types. It applies where animals support the rehabilitation or social care of humans (Kruger and Serpell, 2006). This can involve inclusion of the animals in various activities or a more targeted, pure therapy approach (i.e. a professional using the animal for treatment to heal a specific disorder). This can include post-traumatic stress disorder interventions, such as programmes for soldiers, refugees or those who have suffered traumatic experiences; and support animals for disabled people, such as dogs for the blind or deaf, riding for the disabled, etc. Managed rehoming of animals to people who may benefit from having an animal to care for is also carried out, provided there is a suitable support network, which should include access to support for both the human and animal.
- **Animal-assisted therapy (AAT)**, an AAI where there is a defined goal of directed intervention, in which a trained animal that satisfies certain criteria is an integral part of the treatment process for a particular human client. The process is directed, documented and evaluated by professionals

(Sempik *et al.*, 2010) and the animal, with its handler, becomes part of a treatment plan for a particular patient (Johnson, 2009). This can include assistance animals to help rehabilitate and support those with physical or mental health conditions such as autism, anxiety disorders or attention deficit hyperactivity disorders.

- **Animal-assisted activities (AAA)**, an AAI that may have a therapeutic effect, but is not a true therapy in a strict sense and can include both health personnel or lay persons (Sempik *et al.*, 2010). AAA generally include: non-trained dogs visiting homes for the elderly, hospitals and nursing homes, providing patient support; activities with equines; reading to dogs; petting farms; livestock farming camps, etc.; generic emotional or companion support offered by pets to families, without any direct or specific assistance function as such.
- **Rescue and human support animals**, include programmes where animals are trained to support or rescue humans, such as working dogs or mine detection rats; medical detection and medical alert animals; hearing dogs for the deaf or guide dogs for the blind; laboratory animals supporting the development of research in controlled environments, etc. While some animals benefit or enjoy the training in terms of increased exercise, companionship, etc., there is little information on how animals benefit from these interventions. Further evidence in this area should help to identify true One Welfare interventions.

Animal rehoming can have positive impacts on those benefitting from the animal companionship and on the wider community, by reducing the size of stray cat or dog populations, as well as the number of unwanted animals. This, overall, improves human and societal wellbeing. The value and effectiveness of the animal–human bond in healthy individuals and in animal-assisted interventions are increasingly demonstrated in industrialized countries. However, there are still social and cultural aspects that need to be understood when attempting to increase awareness of animal welfare in this context, and more studies could be done, looking at wider human, animal and societal interactions.

To date there has been considerable anecdotal evidence of the mutual benefits of animal–human interaction (Beck and Katcher, 2003), and some hypothesize that this is due to the clear 'win–win' outcomes observed. For example, in some prison interventions inmates train dogs which would otherwise to be euthanized, allowing them to be adoptable. The dogs get a second chance at a happy life, and the inmates connect with another living being and have the chance to give back to their communities (Wenner, 2012). However, there remains a paucity of evidence (Beck and Katcher, 2003; Johnson, 2009) to demonstrate mutual benefits. More effort to systematically evaluate these types of interventions in terms of benefits to animals, humans (Hosey and Melfi, 2014) and the wider environment is needed.

4.3 Assisted Interventions Involving Animals, Humans and the Environment in Practice

Putting One Welfare aspects of animal and human-assisted programmes into practice requires collaboration between professionals working with humans and animals.

Collaborative approaches will vary according to the assisted intervention programme target group and goals. To align with the One Welfare approach, as a minimum all programmes should include:

- A clear description of the aims and activities of the programme.
- Screening procedures to match humans, animals and a suitable environment (where relevant) to maximize benefits for all.
- Human healthcare professionals able to assess conditions, progress and suitability of programme participants to work with animals.
- Animal professionals able to identify suitable animals for the programme, define care and handling programmes and continuously assess their welfare; where relevant this should also include competent and experienced animal trainers. Veterinary professionals should also be involved, to assess the animals' health, both physical and emotional.
- Environmental professionals who are able to advise on relevant aspects.
- Facilities and resources that enable the programme to run and support participants, including humans and animals, throughout the duration of interventions.
- Collaborative networks that enable extended advice and support within areas not directly addressed by the programme.
- Organizations and institutions managing interventions, where possible, establishing collaborations with a research department that can follow up and help to systematically analyse and record data to contribute to the evidence base in this area.

Ideally, those with experience in the sector would come together to develop guidance on how to measure and analyse interventions so that the evidence base can be compared and gathered globally.

References

Beck, A.M. and Katcher, A.H. (2003) Future directions in human–animal bond. *Research American Behavioral Scientist* 47, 79–93.
Christiansen, S.B., Kristensen, A.T., Sandøe, P. and Lassen, J. (2013) Looking after chronically ill dogs: impacts on the caregiver's life. *Anthrozoos* 25(4), 519–533.
Clower, T.L. and Neaves, T.T. (2015) *The Health Care Cost Savings of Pet Ownership*. Human Animal Bond Research Initiative Foundation, Washington, DC. Available

at: https://habri.org/docs/HABRI_Report_-_Healthcare_Cost_Savings_from_Pet_ Ownership_.pdf (accessed 10 February 2018).

Friedmann, E. and Son, H. (2009) The human–companion animal bond: how humans benefit. *Veterinary Clinics of North America Small Animal Practice* 39(2), 293–326.

Hall, S., Dolling, L., Bristow, K., Fuller, T. and Mills, D.S. (2017) *Companion Animal Economics: The Economic Impact of Companion Animals in the UK*. CABI, Wallingford, UK.

Hosey, G. and Melfi, V. (2014) Human–animal interactions, relationships and bonds: a review and analysis of the literature. *International Journal of Comparative Psychology* 27 (1), 117–142. http://escholarship.org/uc/item/6955n8kd (accessed 21 October 2017).

Hunt, M.G., Bogue, K. and Rohrbaugh, N. (2012) Pet ownership and evacuation prior to Hurricane Irene. *Animals* 2, 529–539.

Johnson, R.A. (2009) Psychosocial and therapeutic aspects of human–animal interaction. In: Rabinowitz, P.M. and Conti, L.A. (eds) *Human–Animal Medicine: Clinical Approaches to Zoonoses, Toxicants and Other Shared Health Risks*. Saunders, Maryland Heights, MD, USA.

Kruger, K.A. and Serpell, J.A. (2006) Animal-assisted interventions in mental health. In: Fine, A.H. (ed.) *Handbook on Animal-Assisted Therapy: Theoretical Foundations and Guidelines for Practice*, 2nd edn. Academic Press, San Diego, CA, USA, pp. 21–38.

Mills, D.S. (2012) One Health – One Welfare: Psychological and physical well-being. Abstract. WSAVA/FECAVA/BSAVA World Congress, 11–15 April 2012, Birmingham, UK. Available at: http://www.vin.com/apputil/content/defaultadv1. aspx?pId=11349&catId=34756&id=5328263&ind=488&objTypeID=17 (accessed 15 October 2017).

Sempik, J., Hine, R. and Wilcox, D. (eds) (2010) Green Care: a conceptual framework. A Report of the Working Group on the Health Benefits of Green Care, COST Action 866, Green Care in Agriculture, Loughborough, UK: Centre for Child and Family Research. Available from: http://www.agrarumweltpaedagogik. ac.at/cms/upload/bilder/green_care_a_conceptual_framework.pdf (accessed 15 October 2017).

Wenner, A. (2012) Prison animal programs: a brief review of the literature. Massachusetts Department of Correction. http://www.mass.gov/eopss/docs/ doc/research-reports/prisonanimalprogramsliteraturereviewfinal.pdf (accessed 15 October 2017).

Section 5

Sustainability: Connections Between Biodiversity, the Environment, Animal Welfare and Human Wellbeing

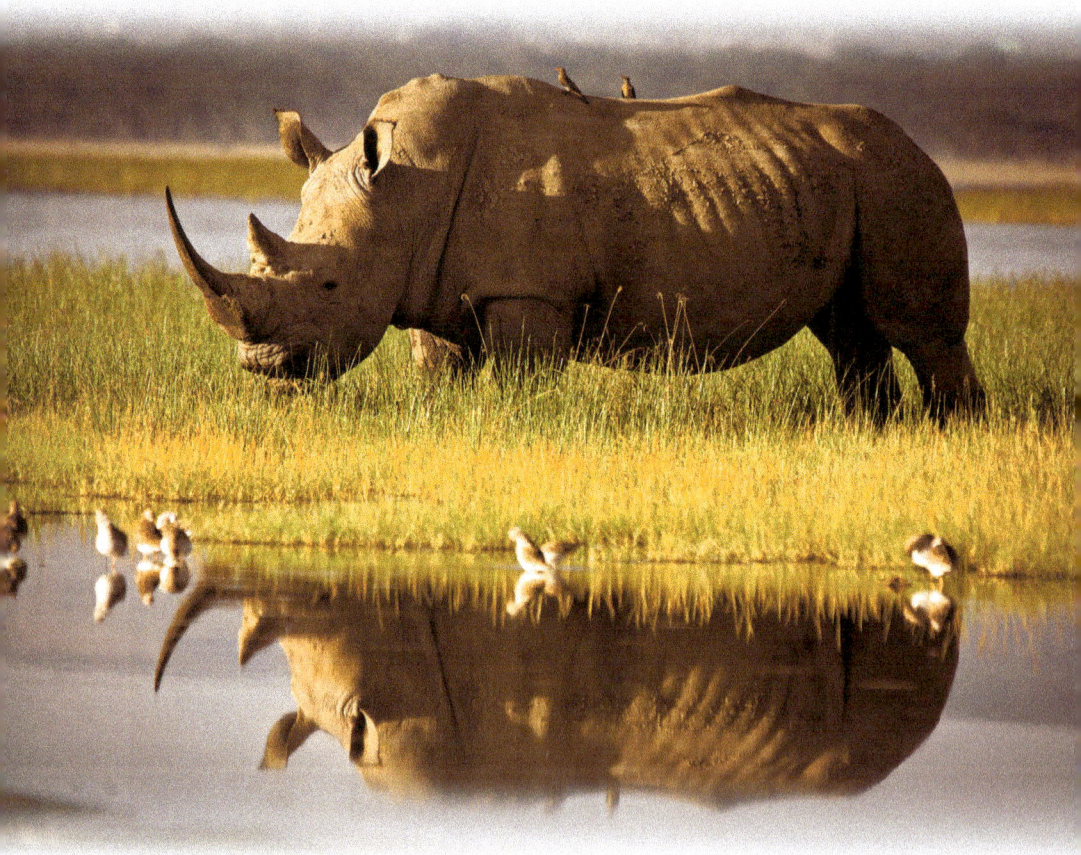

Section 5 of the One Welfare framework explores the links between environmental and conservation issues, animal welfare and human wellbeing. It includes compassionate conservation, aesthetics in the landscape, the impacts of decreased biodiversity, animal–environment conflicts and genetic diversity as support for increased global wellbeing.

There are countless links between animal welfare, human wellbeing, conservation, biodiversity and the environment. This section is closely connected to Section 3; however, it focuses on the wider and more global aspects related to conservation, beyond livestock. Overall it captures important topics relevant for the future success of sustainable development goals across the world that are not fully addressed elsewhere.

Preserving nature is key to the survival of humanity and our planet. Social aspects such as cultural values or the aesthetics of the landscape (e.g. animals as part of the landscape) strongly influence this area. More technical and economic factors are also involved: for example, the decrease in biodiversity and genetic diversity (which will make it difficult to increase food production and productivity worldwide), or the connections between livestock and greenhouse gas emissions and climate change.

Case Study 18 – Building 'Sumak Kawsay' in Equatorial Amazon Kichwa communities (by Arturo Hortas, adapted from Hortas, 2017a,b)

Indigenous people conceive the idea that all beings share the same essence, the same principles of action and the same origin. Based on this principle, we could conclude that we all form part of the same, large community.

The Kichwa villages of Pastaza (Ecuadorian Amazon) consider that the territory they inhabit is fundamental to develop their way of life. In their organization of territorial space there are three principles that govern their worldview:

- *Sumak Allpa* (Land without evil): the living space that a community shares in harmony with nature and the Supai, protective spirits that inhabit it.
- *Sumak Kawsay* (Life in harmony): according to the Amazon Kichwa vision, Sumak Kawsay means life in harmony or life in fullness with all the beings of the *Ayllu*. The *Ayllu* refers to the family, but not only the human family; it also includes all the living beings of the jungle. The *Ayllu* group forms the community and the set of communities, the ancestral villages.
- *Sacha Runa Yachay* (ancestral knowledge): refers to the set of ancestral knowledge that the inhabitants of the *Ayllu* possesses.

To maintain harmony with their environment in a sustainable way and to achieve *Sumak Kawsay* it is paramount to have plenty of vegetation and animals. As part of their lifestyle a forest management system known as *chakra-ushun-purun* is in place; this aims to sustain biodiversity, with a large variety of food, medicine, timber, craft and wildlife.

Testimonies from a member of this community helps us to understand these concepts:

Continued

Case Study 18. Continued.

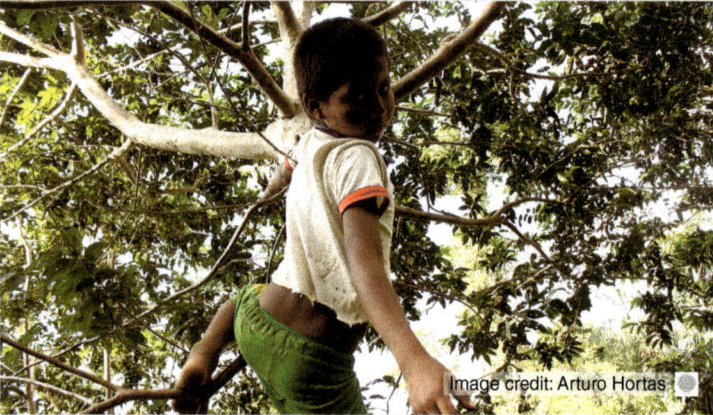

Image credit: Arturo Hortas

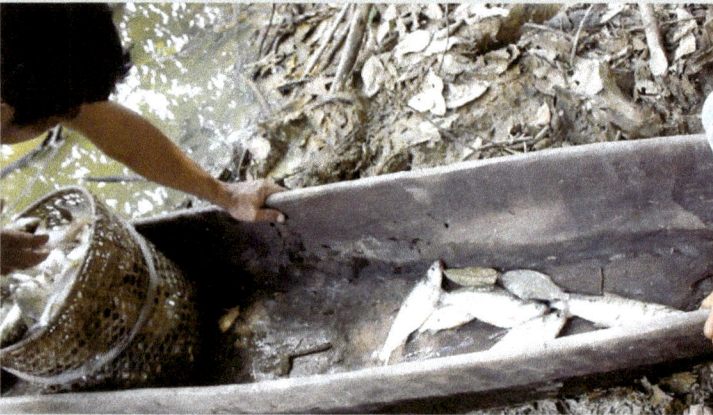

I have sown my crops with all sorts of plants like quilt, camito, ishpingu and pacay. All sorts of animals come around to eat. The satin pig, and the huangana eat from the hearts of palm. Also, armadillos, guantas and guatusas, they all get together to eat from the hearts of palm. Birds like toucans, turkey hens, carunsi, cuisine and paujil.

Another important concept is the *Sumak Yacu*:

Sumak Yacu refers to the biodiversity of all animals that inhabit the waters. It's a river full of lives, or Kawsac Yacu. There are a lot of fish in it, like big catfish. There is also plenty of fish in lakes and streams. It's the home of truly powerful spirits that look after fish and allow them to breed regularly.

The province of Pastaza, within the Ecuadorian Amazon Region, contains a territory named *Kawsak Sacha* (living forest), which covers 140,000 hectares.

Continued

> **Case Study 18. Continued.**
>
> Kichwa nationals live in this region and actively work in the defence of collective and territorial rights, so they can continue building *Sumak Kawsay*.
>
> The *Sumak Kawsay* is an alternative vision to the western economic model, moving away from non-sustainable exploitation of natural resources and focusing on the defence of life in general. It adopts a sustainable lifestyle, aiming to maintain harmony with all living beings in a true One Welfare lifestyle.

The different areas relevant to this section are multiple and interactive. The links between particular changes in ecosystem services and the various indicators of human wellbeing (MA Board, 2005) and animal welfare are often not well understood. However, there are already systems with defined indicators; for example, the Marmot indicators include a diverse range of social, economic and environmental factors and look at the impact on people's health (Marmot Indicators, 2017). Interestingly, animals are not part of that system; yet identifying relevant data correlations between human wellbeing, animals and the environment could help in undertaking a more holistic approach and increase intervention efficiency.

5.1 Interaction Between Diverse Factors

There is an intrinsic connection between biodiversity and ecosystem functions, with multiple areas highly related to other complex factors. This complicates attempts to make statements of causality or to establish the proportionality of various contributors to changes (MA Board, 2005). As an example, it is well established that habitat conversion, degradation and fragmentation of land (usually due to agricultural expansion) and in the oceans (mostly associated with fishing activities) have been the most important direct drivers of biodiversity loss globally in the recent past (MA Board, 2005). This example has obvious connections to: (i) environmental wellbeing; (ii) the welfare of wild and domestic animals losing or having their habitat disturbed; and (iii) local communities who may be losing natural leisure areas or be subject to negative changes within their immediate surroundings, such as increased traffic.

Overall, identifying key indicators that can reflect interactions between the planet's environment, resources and biodiversity including both humans and animals should be a priority.

> **Direct drivers of biodiversity loss globally (MA Board, 2005)**
>
> - **Most important:** habitat conversion (generally for agricultural expansion), degradation and fragmentation.
> - **Increasing impact:** invasive non-native species, nutrient pollution, climate change.

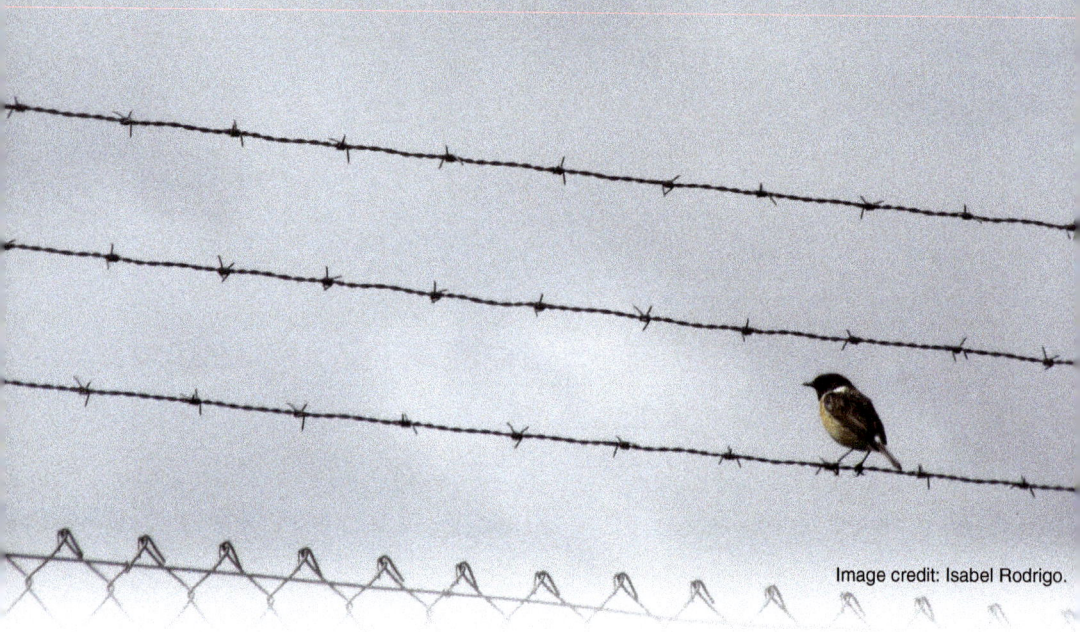

The effects of trade as well as population growth, economic development, and increasing consumption and production together with waste handling are all important indirect drivers of change in ecosystems and ecosystem services. Biodiversity is impacted by the intensification of agriculture, for example by direct biodiversity losses in monocultures, but it is also impacted by intensification due to land fragmentation and loss of habitat (MA Board, 2005). The connections to human, animal and environmental wellbeing cannot be omitted when discussing such matters and future change and policies should aim for a balanced outcome for all. Handling of waste is another indirectly related area.

Discussion and work is already taking place around the conceptual integration of food, sustainability and health management (de Boer and Aiking, 2017), under frameworks such as 'ecological public health'. This principle encourages multidisciplinary work to ensure that public health helps address the entire biological, material, social and cultural dimensions of the human, living and physical world. One Welfare complements this work, aiming to ensure that animal welfare and the wellbeing of people and the planet have an active presence in future work (Lang and Rayner, 2015).

5.2   Conservation and Animal Welfare

Animal welfare (concern mainly for individual animals) and animal conservation (concern mainly for species preservation) have different priorities, and while on first thought the two might seem to be complementary, at times one can be in conflict with the other.

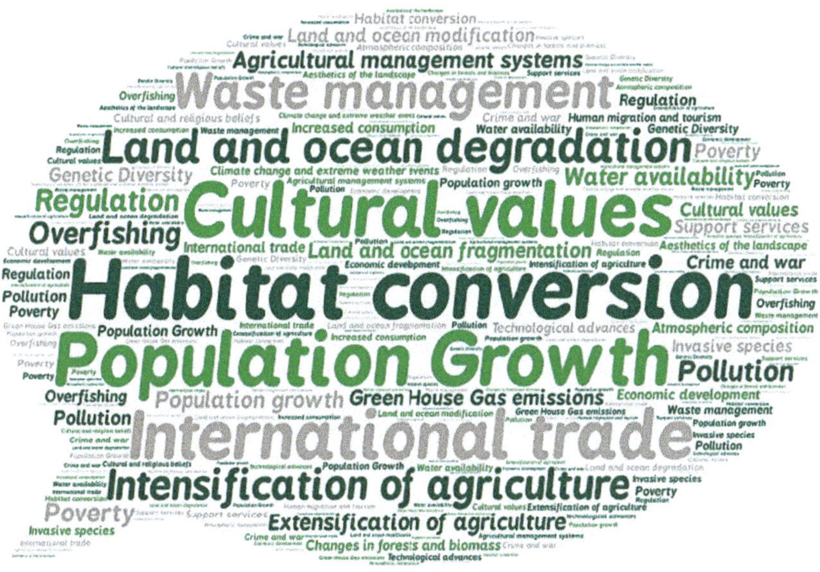

Fig. 5.1. Word cloud of factors that impact One Welfare Section 5.

Some have used the term 'compassionate conservation' to refer to combining the considerations of animal welfare and conservation. The ultimate aim is to use knowledge and techniques from animal welfare science to inform and refine conservation practices. This aims for a reduction in the suffering of individual wild animals, aiming to improve conservation outcomes and to improve stakeholder collaboration and support (Compassionate Conservation, 2017).

Consideration of animal welfare in a conservation context can lead to better conservation outcomes, while engendering increased stakeholder support.

One example that highlights practical conflicts is that as part of conservation strategies animals can be subjected to culling, captivity, relocation and other kinds of constraints on their welfare to support biodiversity. While at times some of these animal welfare issues might be unavoidable for a particular species to survive, or to preserve biodiversity in a particular area, it would be good to identify whether more can be done to improve the welfare of affected animals, acknowledging that animal welfare – including their physical, psychological and social aspects – is critical to preserve biodiversity.

This topic also raises interesting ethical discussions where there might be conflicts between animal and environmental ethicists in considering whether the environments, animals or humans have different values, and whether more effort and care should be taken for one at the expense of others. One Welfare encourages a holistic approach, considering all, and aims to find solutions that provide the best available wellbeing option for all.

An additional issue to consider is the illegal wildlife trade. This impacts on animal welfare, species conservation, ecosystems and local communities. Second to ecosystem loss, illegal trade is the biggest cause of species extinction (HSI and WSPA, 2009). Collaborative efforts to address this alongside other issues are necessary. This element overlaps with some of the socio-economic issues contained in Section 2 of the One Welfare framework, where the connection between animal welfare and crime is discussed.

Case Study 19 – Keeping animals wild: animal welfare for biodiversity and environmental sustainability (by Humane Society International and World Animal Protection)

Illegal wildlife trafficking has a devastating impact on animal welfare, species conservation, ecosystems and the communities that could develop through ecotourism. Second to ecosystem loss, it is the biggest cause of species extinction. Those buying trafficked animals may have little understanding of the damage they are doing to the environment, animals and sustainable development.

Regions with diverse ecosystems may attract wildlife traffickers. In efforts to stem this trade, the governments of several affected countries carry out border inspections where wildlife traffickers are stopped and animals are confiscated.

However, the need for a place to take the animals is often overlooked in confiscation plans. As a result, some regions have lacked the infrastructure necessary to accommodate and ensure the welfare of wildlife confiscated under the Convention on International Trade in Endangered Species of Wild Fauna and Flora (CITES).

As an example, only two countries in one affected region had adequate facilities for wildlife reception and rehabilitation. This means that many of the confiscated but potentially releasable animals are sent to private collections and zoos and spend their lives in captivity.

Education is a preventative element: greater public awareness of the cruelty and environmental damage caused by trafficking is a way to reduce demand, which can in turn reduce poaching. As long as trafficking continues, specialist wildlife rescue centres – housing, treating and rehabilitating confiscated animals in high-welfare conditions – will help ensure the survival of species targeted by traffickers. Successful rehabilitation can lead to reintroduction, helping to reinforce wild populations.

To protect the diversity and welfare of wildlife in affected regions, international animal welfare NGOs have worked closely with local NGO partners, wildlife rescue centres and government departments. Together, they have carried out public education initiatives and assisted high-welfare wildlife rescue centres. The resulting impact is a reduced market for traffickers and increased capacity to care for confiscated wildlife.

In just one affected region, public awareness and education programmes on the trade in illegal wildlife products and exotic pets reached over 500,000 residents

Continued

Case Study 19. Continued.

and tourists in 1 year alone, and rescue centres were able to offer high welfare care for over 1000 animals annually.

Improvements to infrastructure in wildlife centres are ongoing; however, many of the confiscated animals are already being transported safely, fed a balanced diet and rehabilitated, enabling some to be released back into the wild. Wild releases boost the animal populations that encourage ecotourism.

The United Nations[1] recognizes the vital role that education plays in preserving wildlife and the environment by reducing demand for illegal animal products and encouraging local people to protect their natural resources – in this case, the unique wildlife of Central America that attracts so many visitors.

Until this education work has the desired effect, wildlife rescue centres can be supported to provide high welfare care and rehabilitation for confiscated animals. High animal welfare during this period improves the animals' chances of survival and even release, playing a role in maintaining biodiversity through wild populations.

NOTE: This case study has been adapted from the publication 'Keeping animals wild: animal welfare for biodiversity and environmental sustainability' by Humane Society International and World Animal Protection (HSI and WSPA, 2009).

5.3 Air, Land, Water, Climate Change and One Welfare

Animal biodiversity contributes to stable ecosystem services, and extensive livestock rearing maintains carbon sequestration in semi-arid areas. Animals should be much better valued and treated as part of an overall effort to maintain and sustain ecosystem integrity, and thus comprehensive wellbeing (Zinsstag *et al.*, 2015). Integrating the benefits of animal welfare and conservation to conservation agriculture helps to support improvements on a number of aspects such as less labour-intensive production, better management of waste and water availability, and improved soil quality and water filtration. (A video describing an example of conservation agriculture integrating livestock in Southern Brazil can be watched at http://www.fao.org/ag/ca/.)

Responsible animal management can help improve land use. Animals are an important part of the environment and behavioural studies, for example, elucidate the roles of wildlife in biodiversity and ecosystems, and animals' contributions to environmental services (Appleby, 2008).

Changes in forests and biomass impact on atmospheric composition, climate, hydrology, and habitat modification and loss, all of which directly impact animal welfare and human wellbeing. Such changes can increase the risk of landslides, for example, as a result of poor or improved soil retention, or affect trace gases in the atmosphere that subsequently change the chemistry of the troposphere and reduce the atmosphere's capacity to remove pollutants (atmospheric cleansing capacity) (MA Board, 2005).

> **Case Study 20 – Threats to the survival of wildlife: elephants and earthworms (by Peter Stevenson, Compassion in World Farming, CIWF)**
>
> Studies show that population and species extinctions are proceeding rapidly and a sixth mass extinction may already be under way (Ceballos *et al.*, 2017). Human pressures, including agriculture, are an important factor in this. Ever more forests and savannahs are being destroyed to grow soy and cereals for industrially farmed animals. This is eating into wildlife habitats, driving many species – including elephants and jaguars – towards extinction (Lymbery, 2017).
>
> Moreover, the chemical-soaked monocultures that have arisen in part to satisfy the industrial livestock sector's growing demand for feed crops have devastated birds, butterflies and pollinators (Lymbery, 2017). Both the numbers and diversity of earthworms are being reduced by intensive agriculture (Tsiafouli *et al.*, 2015); earthworms are essential to human life as they play a key part in maintaining soil health and fertility.

Animals also impact on other aspects of the environment. There are studies reporting the effect of industrial production on the environment, including pollution of ground and surface water (Mekonnen and Hoekstra, 2012), soil degradation (Edmondson *et al.*, 2014; Tsiafouli, 2015), biodiversity loss (WHO, 2015) and air pollution (Lelieveld *et al.*, 2015). Livestock makes up two-thirds of terrestrial vertebrates by weight, and the study of animal behaviour is helping to develop approaches to management – such as silvopastoral systems – that reduce greenhouse gas production, and air and water pollution, while increasing animal welfare and efficient use of resources (Appleby, 2015; Broom *et al.*, 2013).

While human wellbeing has improved through improved water management by controlling floods, irrigation or generating hydroelectricity (MA Board, 2005), it is important to be mindful of environmental and animal welfare trade-offs for these improvements. These may include habitat fragmentation and loss, biodiversity loss or declines in sediment supplies to the coastal zone (MA Board, 2005). Given that dietary choices and resulting consumption patterns are the drivers of production (Heller *et al.*, 2013) the food we eat is a key driver for change. As a result some have already suggested the adoption of SHARP diets: environmentally Sustainable (S), Healthy (H), Affordable (A), Reliable (R) and Preferred from the consumer's perspective (P) (Mertens *et al.*, 2017).

> The capacity of the oceans to provide fish for food has declined substantially and in some regions shows no sign of recovery (MA Board, 2015).

Changes over the years in fishing, transport and tourism have also had an impact on marine ecosystems. Some might have had a short-lived benefit

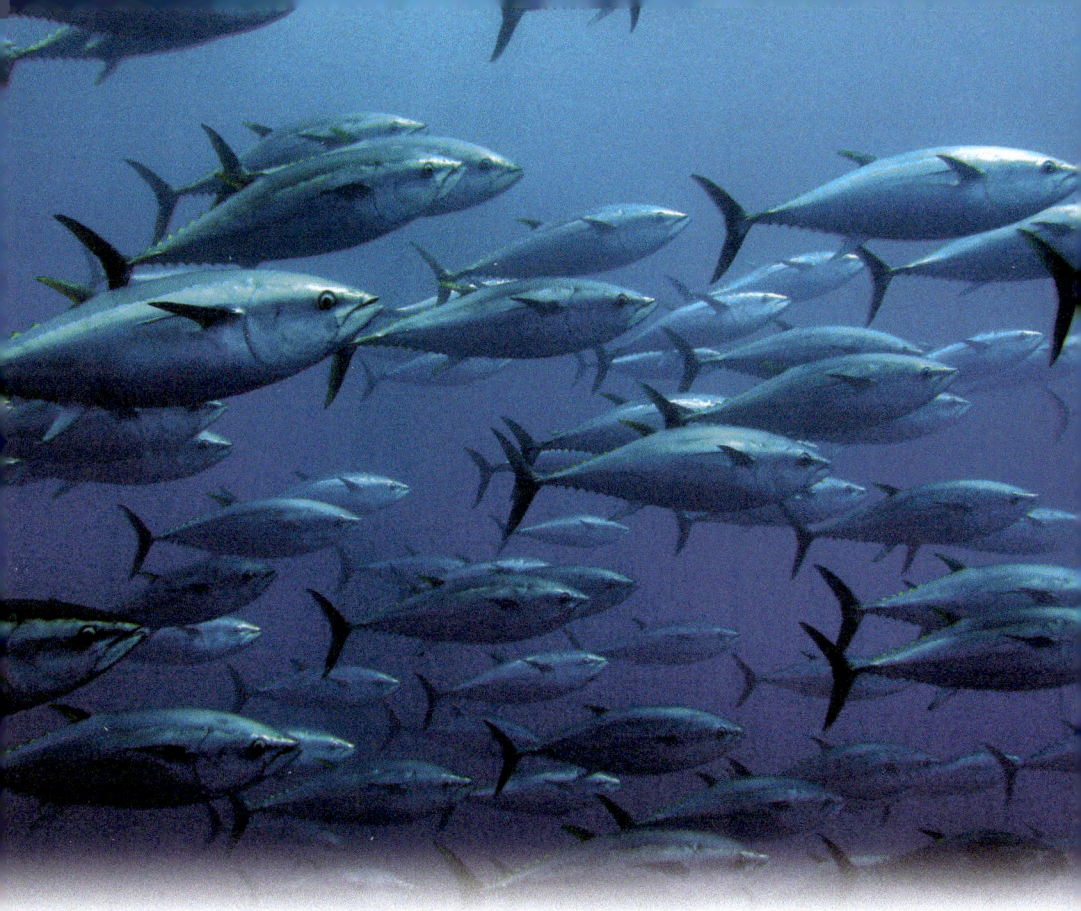

to human wellbeing in terms of increased provision of food from fishing. However, the longer-term picture includes changes from highly diverse, complex and robust coastal ecosystems into systems of reduced diversity and resilience (MA Board, 2005) as a result of overfishing, affecting local communities and resulting in lower wellbeing for all.

Pollution is another global issue that affects animals, humans and the environment. It impacts on everyone's health and wellbeing. Pollution takes many forms, some more easily noticed than others, ranging from plastic and micropollutants in rivers and oceans to poor air quality or industrial waste, litter, light, heat or noise (UN, 2017). The United Nations has identified that interventions to address pollution need to go beyond the environmental sector to include other relevant areas such as agriculture, industry, urban, transport, energy and health (UN, 2017).

Several collaborative multistakeholder platforms are now addressing food security and agriculture issues, for example, and these cover many of the aspects captured in this section. However, it is important for these to interconnect with professionals engaged in animal welfare, conservation, biodiversity, human wellbeing and ecosystems to ensure an inclusive One Welfare approach.

5.4   Biodiversity, the Environment, Animal Welfare and Human Wellbeing in Practice

This is a complex section addressing global topics. How to implement different One Welfare projects or to put in place policies relevant to this section will very much depend on the local area concerned, as well as the specific area of intervention. This relates to the fact that changes in biodiversity and wellbeing are not evenly distributed among individuals, countries or social groups (MA Board, 2005).

The summary below attempts to capture, in very general terms, the basic requirements that may apply to most situations. Those undertaking interventions in this area may, however, identify alternative strategies that help in their specific projects. It might be that prior research work is necessary to identify systematic evaluation tools or indicators that can help to undertake implementation in a consistent way across the world. One example of a systematic evaluation framework tool is the OIE tool for the evaluation of performance of veterinary services (OIE, 2013), which helps assess animal welfare alongside other factors.

The basic requirements may include:

* Aims and objectives of the intervention or programme.
* Identification of all relevant processes and relationships between them in a comprehensive and systematic manner.
* Data and information gathering to document the direct and indirect impacts and trade-offs that need to be considered and addressed.
* Data and information gathering of documented potential interventions and solutions.
* Identification of objective measures that can be monitored to enable assessment of progress.
* Consideration of the minimum capacity needed to achieve an objective that would enable both sustainability and prioritization. Where advanced capacity is unlikely to be developed in the short and medium term, consider available alternatives and what intermediate steps can be taken to build on what exists (STDF, 2016).
* Stakeholder platform including all interested sectors, such as animal welfare, human wellbeing, conservation, biodiversity, ecosystem services, agriculture and livestock or economic growth representatives.

While there seems to be ample evidence on the need for action in this area, wider dissemination of successful solutions is needed. There is a need to integrate and realign policies related to climate, agriculture, food and nutrition (FAO, 2016). Increased sharing of successful One Welfare interventions achieving improvements for humans, animals and the environment is also needed. The creation of a systematic comprehensive system of reporting could help to bring this together and help support global goals.

References

Appleby, M.C. (2008) Animal management and welfare, applied ethology and life as we know it. *Proceedings of the 42nd Congress of the International Society for Applied Ethology*, Ireland, p. 2.

Appleby, M.C. (2015) Applied ethology for ever: animal management and welfare are integral to sustainability. *Proceedings of the 49th Congress of the International Society for Applied Ethology*, Japan, p. 40.

de Boer, J. and Aiking, H. (2017) Pursuing a low meat diet to improve both health and sustainability: How can we use the frames that shape our meals? *Ecological Economics* 142, 238–248.

Broom, D.M., Galindo, F.A. and Murgueitio, E. (2013) Sustainable, efficient livestock production with high biodiversity and good welfare for animals. *Proceedings of the Royal Society of London B* 280(1771), 2013–2025.

Compassionate Conservation (2017) http://compassionateconservation.net/ (accessed 21 October 2017).

Ceballos, G., Ehrlich, P.R. and Dirzo, R. (2017). Biological annihilation via the ongoing sixth mass extinction signaled by vertebrate population losses and declines. *Proceedings of the National Academy of Sciences USA* 114 (30) E6089–E6096. Available at: http://www.pnas.org/content/114/30/E6089 (accessed 16 February 2018).

Edmondson, J.L., Davies, Z.G, Gaston, K.J. and Leake, J.R. (2014) Urban cultivation in allotments maintains soil qualities adversely affected by conventional agriculture. *Journal of Applied Ecology* 51, 880–889.

FAO (2016) The State of food and agriculture, 2016. FAO Publication. Available at: http://www.fao.org/publications/sofa/2016/en/ (accessed 22 October 2017).

Heller, M.C., Keoleian, G.A. and Willett, W.C. (2013) Toward a life cycle-based, diet-level framework for food environmental impact and nutritional quality assessment: A critical review. *Environmental Science & Technology* 47(22), 12632–12647.

Hortas, A. (2017a) Nungulli's daughters. Video. Available at: https://vimeo.com/236724509 (accessed 1 February 2018).

Hortas, A. (2017b) Tsumi, River men. Video. Available at: https://vimeo.com/236725552 (accessed 1 February 2018).

HSI and WSPA (2009) Keeping animals wild: animal welfare for biodiversity and environmental sustainability. HSI and WSPA, London, UK.

Lang, T. and Rayner, G. (2015) Beyond the Golden Era of public health: charting a path from sanitarianism to ecological public health. *Public Health* 129(10), 1369–1382.

Lelieveld, J., Evans, J.S., Fnais, M., Giannadaki, D. and Pozzer, A. (2015) The contribution of outdoor air pollution sources to premature mortality on a global scale. *Nature* 525, 367–371.

Lymbery P. (2017) *Dead Zones: Where the Wild Things Were*. Bloomsbury Publishing, London, UK.

MA Board (2005) Millennium Assessment Board, Ecosystems and Human Wellbeing – Current state and trends assessment. Available at: http://www.millenniumassessment.org/en/Condition.html (accessed 21 October 2017).

Marmot Indicators (2017) Marmot Indicators. Public Health England. Available at: https://fingertips.phe.org.uk/profile-group/marmot (accessed 22 October 2017).

Mekonnen, M.M. and Hoekstra, A.Y. (2012) A global assessment of the water footprint of farm animal products. *Ecosystem* 15(3), 401–415. DOI: 10.1007/s10021-011-9517-8.

Mertens, E., van't Veer, P., Hiddink, G.J., Steijns, J.M. and Kuijsten, A. (2017). Operationalising the health aspects of sustainable diets: A review. *Public Health Nutrition* 20(4), 739–757.

OIE (2013) OIE tool for the evaluation of performance of veterinary services. Available at: http://www.oie.int/fileadmin/Home/eng/Support_to_OIE_Members/pdf/PVS_A_Tool_Final_Edition_2013.pdf (accessed 22 October 2017).

STDF (2016) Joint EIF/STDF: Analysis of consideration given to SPS issues in DTIS. Available at: http://www.standardsfacility.org/stdf-publications (accessed 22 October 2017).

Tsiafouli, M.A., Thébault, E., Sgardelis, S.P. *et al.* (2015) Intensive agriculture reduces soil biodiversity across Europe. *Global Change Biology* 21(2) 973–85.

UN (2017) Towards a Pollution-Free Planet: Background Report. UN Environment Programme, Nairobi, Kenya. Available at: https://wedocs.unep.org/bitstream/handle/20.500.11822/21800/UNEA_towardspollution_long%20version_Web.pdf?sequence=1&isAllowed=y (accessed 10 February 2018).

WHO (2015) *Connecting Global Priorities: Biodiversity and Human Health: A State of Knowledge Review*. WHO Press, Geneva, Switzerland.

Zinsstag, J., Schelling, E., Waltner-Toews, D., Whittaker, M. and Tanner, M. (eds) (2015) *One Health: The Theory and Practice of Integrated Health Approaches*. CAB International, Wallingford, UK.

Index